362.4 Vaughan, C. Edwin
VAU   Social and Cultural
       Perspectives on
       Blindness

DATE DUE

362.4 Vaughan, C. Edwin
VAU   Social and Cultural
       Perspectives on
       Blindness

DATE	ISSUED TO

DEMCO

SOCIAL AND CULTURAL PERSPECTIVES ON BLINDNESS

About the Author

Ed Vaughan received his B.A. degree from West Virginia University and a M.Div. from Union Theological Seminary, New York. He received his M.A. and Ph.D. degrees in Sociology from the University of Minnesota.

For the past twenty-seven years he has been a member of the faculty at the University of Missouri-Columbia. He has served as Chair of the Department of Sociology and as Director of the Center for Research on Aging. He currently holds the rank of Professor in the Department of Sociology at the University of Missouri-Columbia.

In 1991, he was a Visiting Professor at Xi'An Foreign Languages University in the People's Republic of China. He returned in the summers of 1992 and 1994 to continue his research on programs for disabled people in China.

Professor Vaughan has made four trips to various countries in Africa, with additional field work for this book accomplished by his travels in Spain. His earlier book, *The Struggle of Blind People for Self Determination* (1993), reflects his long-term interest in issues related to rehabilitation and blindness in the United States.

SOCIAL AND CULTURAL PERSPECTIVES ON BLINDNESS

Barriers to Community Integration

By

C. EDWIN VAUGHAN, Ph.D.

Professor
Department of Sociology
University of Missouri
Columbia, Missouri

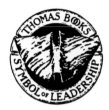

CHARLES C THOMAS • PUBLISHER, LTD.
Springfield • Illinois • U.S.A.

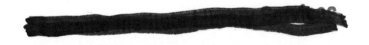

Published and Distributed Throughout the World by

CHARLES C THOMAS • PUBLISHER, LTD.
2600 South First Street
Springfield, Illinois 62794-9265

© *1998 by* CHARLES C THOMAS • PUBLISHER, LTD.
ISBN 0-398-06854-2 (cloth)
ISBN 0-398-06855-0 (paper)

Library of Congress Catalog Card Number: 97-52371

Printed in the United States of America
CR-R-3

Library of Congress Cataloging in Publication Data

Vaughan, C. Edwin.
    Social and cultural perspectives on blindness / by C.
Edwin Vaughan.
        p.   cm.
    Includes bibliographical references and index.
    ISBN 0-398-06854-2 (cloth). -- ISBN 0-398-06855-8 (pbk.)
    1. Blind--Cross-cultural studies. 2. Blind--Education.
3. Blind--Rehabilitation. 4. Blindness--Social aspects.
5. Blindness--Public opinion. I. Title.
HV1593.V36 1998
362.4' 1--dc21   97-52371
                                                                            CIP

For JoAn, Joe, Laura and Stephen
– my great family!

PREFACE

Blindness and rehabilitation programs take many forms in nations and cultures around the world. This book is about these differences and the conditions which produce them. The research is by no means exhaustive. One of the purposes is to help us reflect upon, and not take for granted, ideas and practices about blindness within our own particular cultures.

I could not have completed this research without the assistance of many people. I particularly wish to thank Mr. Aubrey Webson of the Hilton Perkins International Program who helped write Chapter 5, and JoAn Vaughan, Ph.D. from Stephens College who co authored Chapter 4. Gary Wunder, Lawrence Luck, and Marc Maurer kindly prepared special material for this volume.

Numerous individuals in several different countries helped educate me and directly contributed to this work. From Spain, these included Pedro Zurita, Rafael Mondaca, Roberto Garvia, Maria Teresa Carranza Crespo, Consuelo Torres (translator), Jesus Buitrago, and Javier Gutierrez de Tovar. At age 92, Mr. Tovar, the founder of Organización Nacional de Ciegos Españoles (ONCE) in 1938, is still active in the organization.

I wish to thank the many people whom we have met in several African countries, including William Rowland, Gladys Nyaga, Grace Preko, Gertrude Oforiwa Fefoame, Diane Mpiriuwe, Margaret Dir-Baba, and Captain Lamin Seine. I apologize to those many individuals who helped, but are too numerous to mention here.

In the People's Republic of China, I was educated by many blind people, government workers, and ordinary citizens who in 1991 and 1992 did not wish to have their names mentioned. President Sun Tianyi, of the Xi'an Foreign Languages

University, treated me with the greatest kindness and helped make my times in China some of the most memorable in my life. There is no way to mention the many students and faculty who assisted me as guides, translators of documents, and interpreters. I will never forget the many blind people in China who shared with me their personal life experiences.

Those who have contributed to my education in the United States are too numerous to mention. However, several individuals at the University of Missouri Columbia, have helped as readers, research assistants, copy editors, and in other support services. These include Rick Pfeiffer, Felica Beckmann, Diane Rogers, Rita Fleischman, Martin Misiak, Polly Vanamburg, Nikke Berger, Julie Kaplan and Mary Grigsby. My special thanks to Connie Knowles for her patience during several drafts of this manuscript. And a special thanks to my wife, JoAn, who read the entire manuscript and contributed many helpful suggestions.

I wish to acknowledge the support from the Department of Sociology and the College of Arts and Science at the University of Missouri-Columbia. Funding helped support research assistance and travel for field interviews.

Two articles, "Blindness and Managing the Environment" and"Sex Education of Blind Children," which appear in this book were first published in the *Journal of Visual Impairment and Blindness*. They are reprinted with permission from the *Journal of Visual Impairment and Blindness*. Copyright (1987) by the American Foundation for the Blind, 11 Penn Plaza, Suite 300, New York, NY 10001. All rights reserved.

I also thank *The Educator* and *The World Blind* for permission to reproduce selected materials.

This book is a first step, and a halting one at that, toward a comparative study of blindness and social responses to blindness. I am painfully aware of how much more there is to know about the cultures I describe. I hope to continue this research by learning more about blindness in additional cultural regions. Suggestions and corrections are welcome at: Fax - (573) 884-6430 or E-mail - SOCCEV@SHOWME.MISSOURI.EDU.

CONTENTS

Page

Preface   vii

Chapter

1. INTRODUCTION - WHY STUDY REHABILITATION AND   3
   BLINDNESS FROM A CROSS-CULTURAL PERSPECTIVE?

   Point of View   5
   Overview   8
   Politically Correct Language   12
   Summary   15

2. SOCIAL AND CULTURAL PERSPECTIVES ON   17
   BLINDNESS

   Is There A Phenomenological Aspect to Blindness?   17
   Critique of Blindness as a Condition of Existence   20
   Blindness Embedded in Culture   23
   Blindness in a Mexican Village   25
   The Social Context of Blindness   27
   Social Interaction   28
   Organized Services   32
   Blindness and the New World Order   36
   Political Context   39
   Is Blindness Simply a Characteristic?   40
      Blindness: Handicap or Characteristic?   41
      A Characteristic   41
      A Limitation   43
      A Handicap   44
      Alternatives   45
      Services for Blind People   46
      Resignation and Rebellion   47
      Patients or Colleagues?   48
      Active Participation   49

                                                                    Page

3. MANUFACTURING IDEAS ABOUT BLINDNESS   51

    Producing New Images about Blindness   51
    Science as the Highest Form of Knowledge   52
    Blind People as Exotic Objects for Ethnography   53
    Blindness and Consciousness   55
    Blind Racoons   60
    Best Practice   61
    Sample Size and Representativeness   62
    Flawed Use of Research Design   64
    Use of Literature Reviews   65
        Sex Education of Blind Children Re-Examined   67
    Alternatives   69
    Summary   73
    Blindness and Managing the Environment   75
        Subjective Experience and the Environment   76
        Models of the World   77
        Perception Without Sight: A Personal Account   78
        Environmental Modifications   79
        Neoinstitutionalization   86

4. BLINDNESS IN THE UNITED STATES: FROM   89
    ISOLATION TO FULL INCLUSION–*with JoAn Vaughan*

    Cultural Origins of Blindness in Antiquity   89
    Schools for the Blind in the United States   93
    Sheltered Workshops   95
    Agencies and Professions   99
    The Social Context of Agency Development   101
    Workers for the Blind   104
    The Organized Blind   106
    Recent Trends in the Education of Blind Children   108
    Educating Dacia   112
    The Importance of Braille Literacy   113
    Summary   118

5. BLINDNESS IN AFRICA-*with Aubrey Webson*   119

    Prevention fo Blindness   119
    Traditional Views   123
    The Importance of Gender - Sexual Relationships Between   126
        the Blind and the Sighted

Page

International Cooperation 129
Pan-African Cooperation 130
The Gambia 132
From Loss of Sight to Rehabilitation – 134
  One Person's Experience
Uganda 135
Ghana 137
Zambia 138
South Africa 139
Issues of Empowerment in Africa 140
  Empowerment and Human Rights of Blind and 140
  Visually Impaired Persons in Africa

6. BLIND PEOPLE IN THE MIDDLE KINGDOM AND 145
   THE PEOPLE'S REPUBLIC OF CHINA

Ancient China 145
The Modern Era 147
The Rehabilitation Business in China 151
Observing Blindness in China 152
The First Five-Year Plan for People with Disabilities 157
New Laws to Protect People with Disabilities 160
  Education of the Blind in the People's Republic 163
  of China: Attending Classes in Seven Schools for
  the Blind and Meeting Blind Chinese Women (1996)

7. SPAIN'S UNIQUE ORGANIZATION–THE 167
   ORGANIZATION NACIONAL DE CIEGNOS
   ESPANOLES (ONCE)

Historical Background 167
Beginnings of The ONCE 171
A New Occupation: From Begging to Selling Lottery Tickets 172
Goal Displacement 174
Expanding The ONCE's Program for People with 177
  Physical Disabilities
Expanding The ONCE's Business Interests 181
Blind People Taking Care of Themselves 182
The ONCE's Program 183
International Cooperation 187
Summary 189

Bibliography 195
Index 200

SOCIAL AND CULTURAL PERSPECTIVES ON BLINDNESS

Chapter 1

INTRODUCTION
WHY STUDY REHABILITATION AND BLINDNESS FROM A CROSS-CULTURAL PERSPECTIVE?

The last century has witnessed remarkable changes in the life choices available to many women and men who are blind. Some blind people at various places around the world are well employed and are participating as much as they wish in their societies. Others struggle at the very edge of existence, continuing to live by receiving food and shelter from others. In many places, a life of mendicancy is the only way of earning one's bread. Hope abounds, but sometimes reality is brutal. Many blind people can identify with the sentiments reflected in the first paragraph of Dickens's, *A Tale of Two Cities* (1859):

> It was the best of times, it was the worst of times, it was the age of wisdom, it was the age of foolishness, it was the epoch of belief, it was the epoch of incredulity, it was the season of light, it was the season of darkness, it was the spring of hope, it was the winter of despair, we had everything before us, we had nothing before us . . . .

On the one hand, some countries are so economically poor relative to others that almost no public resources are available for the education and rehabilitation of blind people. Even worse, the poorest nations are often those experiencing the highest levels of conflict, where the situation of blind people is even more perilous. On the other hand, some nations, usually the most prosperous, have dedicated significant levels of private and public finances to improve the lives of blind people. In many instances, international and private, nongovernment organizations are sharing their wealth and philosophy about blindness with less economically developed countries. These organizations are transmitting their philosophies and programs to many less developed countries, where they are grafted on to local cultural traditions.

In the midst of all this, some blind people have become active participants in determining their own fates. Many individuals have thought about issues of fairness, justice, human rights, and the full development of their human potential and have created organizations of blind people to pursue common goals. In some countries the organizations are autonomous, well organized, and well financed by blind people themselves. In other places, organizations for blind people are still managed by outside interest groups and professions. Worldwide organizations such as the World Blind Union have emerged as part of the effort to improve economic and social opportunities for blind people.

The results of this ferment vary widely around the world, depending on many conditions including the level of economic development, local cultural traditions about blindness, the particular historical "accidents" of a given country, different degrees of technological advancement, and the emergence of a growing number of well educated blind people who are providing leadership in the struggle for self-determination. This book is about the social origins of these developments. It describes different perspectives regarding blindness and the social arrangements created for and by blind people. The viewpoints of blind people themselves receive prominent attention in this book.

Blind and visually impaired people are as varied in their human qualities as the rest of the population. Even without blindness, some of them would no doubt fail in society. Like sighted individuals, many have been successful despite obstacles, some have become totally dependent on the welfare state and are content, while others have become inured to the worst definitions of what it means to be blind in any society.

Even within a given nation, blind people as both individuals and as groups differ from each other because they have different personal histories and may represent different cultural or ethnic traditions. It is impossible to generalize about blind people. However, it is a human tendency to have stereotyped views about blindness in any particular culture. Citizens, in general, and professionals who provide education and rehabilitation services usually view blindness ethnocentrically: they judge practices of other cultures from their own vantage point. Preoccupied with our own traditions, programs, organizations, and institutions, we often fail to see the wide array of social and cultural arrangements involving blind people in other societies. A central idea of this book is that blindness itself results in no particular social arrangements or cultural patterns. People are socialized to expect ideas about appropriate behavior for blind people and these expectations vary from culture to culture around the world. It is my hope that education and rehabilitation practices will be enriched as we learn more about blindness from cross-national and cross-cultural perspectives.

POINT OF VIEW

This book in a very limited way describes blindness in four different cultures. My sources are my own firsthand observations as an outsider visiting them, interviews and written material. Much can be learned in almost every country concerning innovative ways in which blind people participate in their societies. Many European countries have well-funded programs with long traditions. Future comparative research should also explore blindness in Islamic regions. There are also important developments in several Asian countries other than China. I look forward to collaborating with others to develop a more complete cross-cultural understanding of blindness and related patterns of education, rehabilitation, and employment.

In most cases, my information is taken from what I call the "organized" blind. In these cultures, organizations of blind people cooperate, in varying ways, to improve their economic and social positions and to move from tutelage to self-determination. Leaders and social movement members neither speak for nor represent all blind people. However, they do tend to be in positions that enable them to be more knowledgeable about social conditions than isolated individuals. Whenever possible, I have included the opinions of ordinary rank and file blind people—those who have solved the everyday problems of living. I have spent considerable time in the People's Republic of China and have made six trips to the regions of Africa described in Chapter

5, and I have firsthand contact with the dominant organization of blind people in Spain. I am not an expert on these cultures, but I think I have been successful in finding reliable people to review this material.

As a sociologist, I am interested in patterns of education, rehabilitation service, socialization, and ideas about blindness. My focus is on the bureaucratic structure of agencies that provide services. Many of these agencies and programs are well established, well funded, and dominated by professionals possessing definite opinions about the needs of blind people. In some countries, the programs are in the earliest stages of development. My greatest interest, however, lies in the social consequences which result when nongovernment organizations, usually groups of well funded citizens of formal colonializing nations, transport their ideas and practices to more traditional and less economically developed societies. I also investigate the economic interests of professional groups that frequently result in patterns of domination and subordination. In *Economy and Society*, Max Weber (1951, 2:943) analyzed the role of social structures in patterns of social domination. Domination may be but is not exclusively pursued for economic advantage. According to Weber, it works best when those who are dominated pursue their interests within a narrow range of opportunities forced upon them by external circumstances. Government officials, agency personnel, professionals, consultants, and so on, benefit both economically and in terms of social status by organizing and otherwise providing educational rehabilitation programs that come to be seen as opportunities by blind people. Patterns of domination are most stable in a closed market; seldom does a blind person have alternatives. This situation becomes even more morally reprehensible if the programs result in dependency on the agency itself, rather than autonomy and independent living. Weber provides a theoretical framework that makes the concept of social control central to analysis of patterns of socialization, to all types of social arrangements whether considered normal or anomalous.

Although I am a sociologist, I am not a disinterested observer. At age sixteen, forty-three years ago, I experienced vision loss which led to my first encounter with the rehabilitation system. The counselors and testers I met recommended that I consider going to college, and the state of West Virginia through its rehabilitation program paid a small part of the cost. For the next twenty-five years, my education continued and my career as a sociologist developed. I gave little thought to blindness, except insofar as it was occasionally a personal nuisance to me. I experienced feelings ranging from annoyance, to humor, to anger when encountering discrimination or inappropriate social behavior relating to my blindness. In 1978, an acquaintance invited me to attend an annual meeting of the National Federation of the Blind. I was struck by the philosophy about blindness being expressed by many speakers, the vigor of the organization, and the commitment to share with the public a more positive view of blindness, the promotion of employment opportunities, and its opposition to discrimination. For me, the five-day meeting was an introduction into a dynamic social movement. After this first encounter, I wanted to learn more, not only because of my personal history, but also because I am a sociologist. For the past decade much of my research and writing has focused on blindness and related issues. I have studied both the organizations of blind people and the social origins of conflict between them and those of professional service providers. The limited views I have often encountered have convinced me of the importance of broader, cross-cultural perspectives on blindness.

This book is critical in its perspective. My purpose is to analyze patterns of domination and subordination as they take various forms in different cultures. I am opposed to social inequality based on gender, ethnicity, or physical condition. Many blind people have had their lives unnecessarily restricted in the name of benevolence, while their benefactors have advanced their careers, increased their social prestige, and gained control of economic resources. While none of these undesirable conditions occur everywhere education and rehabilitation service are offered, they occur frequently enough. Poorly informed people, both sighted and blind, have advanced their careers by creating social arrangements and ideas about blindness that result in unnecessary dependence. Many agencies and programs themselves become barriers in the way of blind people who hope to participate fully in their societies.

I earlier mentioned that the point of view of blind people is central to this book. I share this experience and perspective. However, sighted people, as such, are not excluded from the social movement to provide equal opportunity for blind people. To be helpful, using Irving Goffman's term, they must become "wise." There are sympathetic sighted people willing to share blind peoples' point of view and interact on terms of equality and mutual respect (Vaughan 1993, p. 29). The only basis of cooperation is mutual respect. When differences persist, the perspective emerging from organizations of blind people must be paramount. No one has a monopoly on knowledge, but organizations of blind people reflect the opinions of those most immersed in the experience of blindness. These individuals and their organizations are as rational and intelligent as anyone else and, while appreciating opinions from other perspectives, have the right of self determination.

OVERVIEW

Chapter 2 presents a distinct point of view about the human condition usually labeled "blindness" or "visual impairment." The chapter asks, "Is any particular form of social behavior inherent in blindness itself? Does blindness make people different in irrevocable and important ways from other humans?" Behavior associated with blindness is embedded in all cultures. We are so immersed in our own culture that we seldom have opportunities to be aware of the many different behaviors that blind people can both create and learn in other societies. In this chapter I question the argument that there is a phenomenology of blindness. I discuss the concept of "culture" and describe several aspects of blindness in a Mexican village. Not only cultural traditions, but levels of economic development are important variables for understanding many aspects of the world experienced by blind people. Culture here includes all that we know and all the things we make, including social arrangements and organized activities. The location or situation we occupy in a particular culture is also important. Some societies develop elaborate programs and institutions to educate, rehabilitate, and sometimes employ blind people. Unfortunately, these sometimes become barriers to full participation in a community. When a person is blind or becomes blind, he or she faces new conditions which frequently result in altered relationships with others. The individual has much to learn and is suddenly confronted by parents, friends, teachers, and service providers who may have widely different ideas about blindness and future prospects available to blind people. Organized responses to blindness vary from culture to culture, but most depend on available economic resources.

In many cases, models of education and rehabilitation services are being transported from richer to poorer nations. There is pressure from international organizations to promote generalized services that, I argue, can be harmful. National policies related to disability programs may expand or contract with the economic or political fortunes of a given society. Dramatic examples are described in later chapters dealing with the People's Republic of China and Spain. Blind people themselves sometimes create large organizations, become active in the political process, and address issues of interest to blind people themselves. They usually focus on unfair social conditions and unequal social relationships. In every society, images about blindness are being continually produced, and many people earn their livelihoods by intentionally creating new ideas about blindness. These are usually high status individuals such as published authors or professionals doing scholarly research, who create symbols justifying patterns of domination and subordination. While many argue that blind people have unique problems that require the specialized knowledge of professionals, in many cases blind people themselves reject the new images and their domination by organizations judged to be paternalistic and exploitative.

In Chapter 3, I examine the idea that in an affluent society, science is often considered the highest or most correct source of knowledge. I review several examples of how professionals, using the aura of science, put forth ideas that contribute to false stereotypes about blindness. I also analyze the uncritical use of scientific methodology. It is often assumed that numbers represent hard facts that are free from subjective ideas and that the usual norms that guide scientific research be followed. I argue that interdisciplinary approaches be stressed to minimize the biases of a narrowly focused field dedicated to providing services to blind people and I suggest several ways research can be empirical. Finally, I find that comparative research, cross-cultural research case studies, historical research, and qualitative research are better avenues to understanding blindness.

In Chapter 4, I examine the environments of special education, rehabilitation, and employment programs. The United States is a relatively prosperous nation and large amounts of both private and government money have been spent to improve the condition of blind people. This chapter illustrates that many programs and traditions in the United States were greatly influenced by education and rehabilitation efforts already existing in Europe. In fact, some European institutional arrangements and organizational patterns had previously developed in ancient Greece. Western religious traditions have for more than a thousand years contributed to social arrangements created for blind people. Schools for blind children developed in the United States as early as 1832, and were modeled directly from schools that had existed for several decades in most European countries. Through the leadership of Samuel Gridley Howe, who spent a year studying schools in Europe before accepting his leadership position, Perkins School for the Blind emerged as the national leader. Several other schools appeared in this decade and usually developed with similar philosophies and programs, such as vocational instruction as a means of preparing students for outside employment.

During the nineteenth century, employment opportunities were few and many schools added sheltered workshops. These were also influenced by several different European cultural traditions, and were gradually separated from schools. The chapter describes the rapid development of private agencies, a national organization of educators, and a separate organization of "Workers for the Blind" at the beginning of the twentieth century. Following World War I, revenues from national government sources were made available, thus initiating a period of continuous growth in both federal and state programs. Another important influence was the beginning of the nationally funded Social Security system in 1935. Policies and programs for blind people now had to be considered at the national level. In this context, several state organizations came together in 1940 to become the National Federation of the Blind. Self determination has characterized the ongoing efforts of this Federation and it has emerged as the most influential organization of blind people in the United States.

In Chapter 5, I describe aspects of blindness that are more dominant in less economically developed countries. I recognize the cultural and geographic diversity of the African continent, and select some of the most important features of blindness in sub-Saharan Africa. This chapter begins by stressing the importance of prevention programs being used to reduce the high prevalence rates of blindness. The issue of gender and blindness exists in every culture, but the consequences for women are most evident in those with relatively low levels of economic development. I also consider some of the problems which result when Western models of special education and rehabilitation services are exported to and grafted onto traditional societies. Although many countries could have been selected for special attention, I chose Uganda because of some of its recent political and economic developments and the rapid development of its Organization of the Blind. The chapter examines some views about blindness and physical disability that are features of different ethnic cultural traditions. The rapidly growing number of leaders and organizations of blind people auger well for future generations of blind people in Africa.

In Chapter 6, I discuss China because it has the longest continuous cultural and social history of any contemporary nation. Early on, blind individuals became prominent for their contributions to various emperors in several dynasties. They formed guilds where massage, fortune telling, story telling, music, and begging were widely recognized sources of income. There is evidence that these guilds were autonomous and managed by blind people themselves, for China had neither the humanistic nor "nobless oblige" traditions of the West that created special institutions to take care of blind people. However, there were a few blind schools created under Christian missionary auspices. With the establishment of the People's Republic of China in 1949, autonomous or independent organizations were no longer permitted by the centralized state and the guilds of blind workers disappeared. Many of their traditional occupations were considered backward and inappropriate in a modern socialist state. But in 1978, China began to modernize and become open to outside influence with the ascendancy of Deng Xiao Ping. His son, Deng Pu Fang, emerged as the leader of a government-dominated organization for disabled people. The chapter describes the changing fortunes of blind people during this period, particularly through the impact of the free market economy which has become a significant feature of modern China in the last two decades. This chapter also describes China's first Five Year Plan for disabled people and the appearance of new laws to improve their cause.

In Chapter 7, I describe a unique Spanish organization of blind people which has been more successful than any other at providing employment opportunities and relatively high levels of earned income. Authorized by General Franco in 1938 near the end of the Spanish Civil War, this small organization brought together the many informal groups of blind people. The Organization National Ciego

España (ONCE), has flourished and become one of the leading enterprises of modern Spain, where blind people have a lower unemployment rate than sighted people. The ONCE workers, at the entry level, are guaranteed more than twice the national minimum wage. Here blind people are not welfare clients of the state, but proud employees in their own organization. Acquiring additional businesses to broaden its economic base and to provide a wider array of employment opportunities, the ONCE has now broadened its umbrella to include people with other disabilities. The money generated by this organization helps strengthen the World Blind Union and many countries whose linguistic and cultural traditions are related to Spain.

POLITICALLY CORRECT LANGUAGE

Several readers will have already noticed that I do not follow the politically correct language of blindness required by many government documents in the United States and preferred by many educators and professionals. Proponents would have everyone use people-first language, such as "people who are blind" rather than "blind people" or "a person who is deaf" rather than "a deaf person." By so doing they claim to focus on the whole person rather than the disability. In April, 1993, an agency executive, expressing his concern for uniform usage, wrote to Dr. Kenneth Jernigan, President Emeritus of the National Federation of the Blind, "The point is that the language is now putting people first rather than our disability." He went on to say that there had been agreement about this in the Independent Living movement for several years.

In that same month, in a meeting of the editorial board of a major journal of which I am a member, a prominent educator argued that the blindness field should "get on with it." I have also received specific instruction from journal editors to use the preferred language—"people who are blind." I regret to say that I have sometimes acquiesced in order to get an article past the gatekeepers. The issue has become so important to some that it has even led to empirical research published in major journals.

One of the most recent is an article by Jan La Forge (1991) which tabulated the use of preferred language in all major articles in three major rehabilitation journals in 1988 (p. 50). She concluded that, despite fifteen years of professional effort, preferred language is used only about 50 percent of the time (p. 50). "Perhaps those of us in the rehabilitation profession may need to confront our own possible limiting attitudes before we are enabled to lead the public in consistently employing language signifying positive regard for all humankind–including those with disabilities" (p. 51). Using the preferred language –persons first–puts the so-called correct user on the side of humanity and human rights–surely a good place to be. However, near the end of her research, she includes what I judge to be a crucial observation: "We do not even have data to support the claim, and belief, that those who are disabled themselves prefer what is now called non-disabling language" (p. 51). Most of the arguments I have encountered are put forward by the proponents of preferred language, who are so immersed in their crusade that they do not even demonstrate an awareness of other points of view.

Sometimes preferred language is rejected for literary reasons; it is awkward, tiresome, and repetitive and it makes articles needlessly long. Reading repetitions of the phrases "persons who are blind" or "people who are visually impaired" becomes tiresome to anyone after ten to fifteen occurrences. This criticism is certainly on the mark; however, it is the least significant of the arguments against the preferred language crusade.

I wonder if the proponents of people-first language believe that putting disabled people first on the printed page accomplishes anything in the real world? Does it alter attitudes, professional or otherwise, about disabilities? What is their evidence? The awkwardness of the preferred language calls attention to a person as having some type of "marred identity" (Goffman, 1963).

There are at least two ways to look at this issue. First, the awkwardness of the preferred language focuses on the disability in a new and potentially negative way. In common usage, positive pronouns usually precede nouns. We do not say, "people who are beautiful," "people who are handsome," "people who are intelligent," etc. Under the guise of the preferred language crusade, we have focused on disability in an ungainly new way but have done nothing to educate anyone or change anyone's attitudes.

Second, we are told that preferred usage will cause us to focus on the whole person. In the best of all possible worlds, where ignorance, stereotypes, and advantages over others do not exist, this might be the case. But until we reach that condition—and that will be a long time coming—might it not be preferable to use language that reflects the actual experiences of most disabled people? In interaction with others, disabilities are almost never ignored. Disabled people learn to manage such situations. If we are going to expend this concentrated effort, why not launch a broader-based, more substantive crusade which would change images and ideas about conditions that are sometimes frightening and seldom well understood? For example, why not work on changing the connotations of what it means to be blind—to challenge old understandings with new insights about blindness? Many blind people are proud of the accomplishments of their brothers and sisters. Just as black became beautiful, blind is no longer a symbol of shame. To say, "I am blind" or "I am a blind person" no longer seems negative to many, particularly those groups with existential interest in the topic.

Finally, in the broadest sense, this issue is a political one. From the first book of the Judeo/Christian Bible to the work of Michel Foucault, giving a name is important and suggests domination (Vaughan, 1993, pp. 115-142). There are many different kinds of people with various disabilities. Some groups may have progressed more than others in their effort to redefine their situations in the wider society. Some individuals and groups of individuals wish to name themselves (or at least not have new labels, preferred usage, created for them by "experts"). So why the current people-first language crusade? Why not respect the wishes and diversity of many directly involved individuals and consumer groups? Is this not in part what empowerment is about? No one objects to other people's use of awkward phrases such as "persons with blindness," if they want to be tedious writers. But isn't it pretentious to make such convolutions the preferred or even the only acceptable constructions? Is this not rather the effort of some misguided professionals who, without listening, are trying to change the world of those they purport to serve?

I know that many well-meaning professionals will disagree and wonder how anyone could question the benevolence of the preferred language crusaders. To me, however, this is a measure of their isolation from the very thinking and actions within disability groups that hold the greatest prospect for changing attitudes and behavior. The concept of preferred language is merely academic—in the worst sense

of the term. It means very little with respect to anything of consequence in the everyday world. Whenever I have tried to explain this
issue to blind acquaintances living in other cultures, the only consistent response is amusement.

SUMMARY

It is my hope that this book will contribute to sociology in the areas
of social control and the study of behavior that is considered deviant
or different. I also hope to stimulate interest in cross-national and cross
cultural studies of blindness or disability. I hope that this book makes
a contribution to the growth of a broader perspective for those who
provide education and rehabilitation services. Finally, it may make a
contribution to those blind people who are reflective about their own
situation and are working to make it better.

Chapter 2

SOCIAL AND CULTURAL PERSPECTIVES ON BLINDNESS

Do all blind people have something in common resulting from their lack of vision? Does blindness make them different in irrevocable and important ways from other humans? Are experiences derived from blindness different from other experiences in life? Is there a phenomenology of blindness? In this chapter, I will argue that there is no basic experience which all blind people must confront, and propose instead that blindness is a culturally created phenomenon. Next, I will describe the lives of the blind in a Mexican village and contrast it with those in more economically developed societies. After discussing the cultural context of blindness, I will conclude this chapter with a review of the major types of organized responses to blindness and the political context of rehabilitation programs.

IS THERE A PHENOMENOLOGICAL ASPECT TO BLINDNESS?

William Rowland, who lives and works in South Africa, describes the problem as follows: "Here the aim is to describe blindness as *pure experience*—not what it appears to be to the outside observer, but what it subjectively is in terms of lived-through situations" (p. xiv). Rowland's analysis pertains only to people who have no residual vision: those who are congenitally blind. In fact, he considers the differences between congenitally and adventitiously blind people to be unbridgeable. Adventitiously blind and partially-sighted people have different phenomenological experiences: they have either experi-

17

enced vision or have some degree of vision. According to Rowland, to
be blind means to have experiences of a certain kind and to be
engaged in or disengaged from the world in a certain way.

Rowland asks, "What is it like to be blind?" He wishes to suspend or
eliminate from consideration the attitudes of those who provide services to blind people and several different theoretical perspectives
which have been developed to explain blindness: for example,
Blindness Under Sexual Innuendo, Blindness as Death/Rebirth,
Blindness as the Loss of Consciousness, Blindness as the
Reprogramming of the System, Blindness as a Personal Characteristic,
and Blindness as the Learned Social Role (pp. 14-31). Suspending or
eliminating previous interpretations, he thinks, enables us to better
understand the basic phenomenological experience of blindness.
"Certainly, blind people are frequently the subject of observation and
inductive science, but in the present instance, the insight has to come
from a consideration of the *individual situation* and the *illuminating
example* taken from personal experience" (p. 45). Moreover, he claims
that autobiographical accounts have special significance because they
can be applied universally.

Rowland's method is to analyze the reoccurring elements in the
lives of blind people. At any point in a blind person's life, subsequent
events are influenced by blindness. Blindness usually involves an
accumulation of disappointing experiences and uncertainty about the
future (p. 47). Rowland presents five case studies in which disappointment and uncertainty are chief characteristics. However, he does conclude his discussion by observing that the experience of blindness is
not always negative. A blind man may experience intense feelings of
pride at his graduation ceremony or after being appointed to an influential position. Rowland's two positive examples achieve success in
spite of blindness, while his five negative ones encounter disappointment in lives which are thought to have gone awry because of blindness.

Next, Rowland contrasts the ways in which blind and sighted people experience the world. For most people, sight is the primary sensory mode because it tends to dominate other avenues of perception. "In
contrast to perception with sight, the perception of the blind person is
characterized by fluctuating dominance, the primary interplay being
between touch and hearing" (p. 51). Because the blind person's perception is partial, he or she faces what Rowland calls the threat of "per-

ceptual poverty." "It is overcome through imaginative enrichment of the sensory information. The blind person is able to supplement that which he hears, feels, or perceives in any other way by drawing upon descriptions given by sighted people" (p. 52).

The various senses present our environments in differing degrees. Touch is immediate, while hearing and vision come to us from afar. If the blind person is not to be limited by his reduced horizons, he must actively pursue sensory information, and he enriches his perception from memory and the assistance of others.

For Rowland, blindness also results in linguistic differences.

> Generally, we propose to distinguish between two forms of verbalism: a.) empty usage, where the blind person cannot have direct sensory awareness of the objects or phenomena in question; and b.) vague usage, where, because of a lack of opportunity or personal initiative, the blind person has only a vague or modified conception of the objects and phenomena in question. (p. 55).

He concludes that blind people can have no conception of colors. "Colors cannot be perceived through any of the senses except sight, and so must forever be mysterious to the blind, it is reasoned" (p. 55). Yet blind people, through their initiative, can enrich their understanding. For example, a sighted person cannot see x-rays, but can understand the concept through verbal explanations.

According to Rowland, "Social intercourse has a perceptual foundation. Therefore, the sparseness of information and the lack of giveness that characterize the perception of blind people have a profound effect in the formation of their human relationships" (p. 60). The author discusses these relations in the context of a man's relationship to his family. In his example, contrary to his stated focus on the congenitally blind, Rowland describes a man who suddenly becomes blind. For this man, all relationships go awry, while the sighted person does more of the household work and experiences more stress.

According to Rowland, blind people live in a state of "beholdedness," a perspective requiring assistance in reading, transportation, and shopping. "Now it might be said that every human being sometimes requires help in tackling a tricky problem or facing a ticklish situation. This is true, but the blind person is justifiably sensitive about the help he receives because of the variety of his needs and, particularly because he has no choice" (p. 64).

The blind person may also experience a decline in self-respect, and inequality usually results. Rowland argues that blind people experience reduced options because of necessary "collectivization." They may go to schools for the blind, training centers for the blind, workshops and social organizations for the blind. Others in the society then see these social organizations as the places where blind people ought to go. "It is as if there were a system manufacturing personal histories according to a set design" (p. 66). Eventually, a social welfare system, funded by government resources and charitable contributions, develops to take care of blind people.

CRITIQUE OF BLINDNESS AS A CONDITION OF EXISTENCE

Rowland's attempt to describe blindness "as it is in itself" (p. 44), freed from theoretical explanations of blindness and from the received traditions of professionals and others who provide services to blind people is commendable. So, too, is his effort to distinguish what is to be regarded as the result of blindness as such, and what is to be regarded as the effect of nurture and circumstances. "To be blind likewise means to have experiences of a certain kind and to be engaged in, or disengaged from, the world in a certain way" (p. 44). Although I have great respect for Mr. Rowland as a scholar and leader of the South African Society for the Blind, I think he makes a serious mistake when he denies the importance of culture in his study.

I have quoted Rowland's approach at some length in an effort to present his argument fairly. However, I first question his most basic assumptions about the consequences of being unable to experience the world visually. My argument is based on countless discussions with blind people over the past 40 years, and on my reading of a considerable amount of literature written by blind people, mostly by blind people from the United States. While I have met many and read much by people with experiences and sentiments similar to those described by Rowland, I have met at least as many, and I think more, who have had different experiences and sentiments. My own curiosity has focused most on people who have no residual vision. Contrary to the notion of a single, essential experience of blindness, I have found such a wide variety of descriptions that it would be difficult to explain the wide variability observed and I must question some of the particular social consequences of blindness that Rowland relates.

Because blind people lack visual stimulation, some writers have argued that they experience less of "reality." But in this context, what is reality? Whatever it is, its philosophical and humanistic depths have not been plumbed by visual acuity. If I may be permitted to stretch an analogy, all languages are equally useful to members of various societies. Similarly, any consistently used and well understood means of exploring one's world may be equally useful, whether for blind people, deaf people, or any other group with a particular physical characteristic. Not being able to see stars or clouds does not mean that individuals will have negative reactions to life's experiences. Rowland does observe that much can be learned through alternate means, but his case studies, with two exceptions, describe negative reactions. Why should the assumption be made that something never experienced visually will necessarily produce feelings of essential disappointment (p. 47). I know many congenitally blind individuals for whom this is not true.

This brings the discussion to one of my central assumptions: there is no inherent meaning in any experience. We always learn from our own particular culture the meaning or usage of the symbolic language we use to analyze our experience. We also frequently acquire from our culture positive or negative sentiments associated with different conditions. The absence of visual perception results in no particular symbolic understanding or emotional feelings. These are always acquired from others, from our earliest moments of socialization or, perhaps, from our newly encountered experience with blindness.

In what appears to be an overstatement, Rowland argues that colors cannot be experienced. Again, I can only remind readers that many blind people experience colors in various ways, ranging from heat, texture, and descriptions learned from other people. What is learned is significant to the blind person: heat of the sun may be felt as red, while ice may be felt as some other color associated with coldness. At the end of this chapter, I have included the article, "What Color is the Sun?" which describes a blind mother's efforts to communicate her understanding of the experience of color to her daughter.

Rowland thinks blindness has certain consequences in relationships, which he illustrates using vignettes from family life. However, all of his examples come from middle class families living in industrial urban societies. As I will show later in this chapter, blindness exists in quite diverse cultural and economic settings which determine how blindness is understood and, subsequently, how relationships are affected. For example, relations may not be more complicated if the blind person in a family is extremely wealthy or if other members value attributes associated with blindness.

Scholars are still publishing articles claiming to analyze the basic experience of blindness. Recently, Billington and Karlsson (1997) published what they call a psychological, philosophical, phenomenological analysis of aspects of blindness based on interviews with ten blind people in Sweden. Incidentally, of the ten subjects, three were not congenitally blind. The subjects had previously taken part in related research and in an unspecified way were recruited "through a national organization for blind persons" (p. 153). "The aim of this qualitative-interpretive, phenomenological - psychological study was to discover the essential dimensions (distinctive features) of the body experiences of congenitally blind people" (p. 151). the authors attempt to anchor their work in Hussesl's phenomenological approach to philosophy, which will help explicate the "meaning structure" of a person's statements about experiences. These authors think that the material will "speak for itself." The researcher brings no preconceptions to the analysis.

Quickly abandoning the philosophical jargon, they jump to what would appear not to be a phenomenological starting point. "Training for body awareness is especially important for children who are blind, who learn early to be careful, which contributes to their inhibitions about spontaneous movement and touching others in social situations" (pp. 151 152).

The authors claim that the subjects remember how, as children, they were taught to behave properly. This is a problem, believe it or not, because they are blind. "For people who are blind, the objectification of the body presents a special difficulty in that it is accomplished, for the most part, through the visual sense. Blind persons cannot objectify the bodies of others in the same way that sighted persons can objectify blind persons' bodies" (p. 157). Such insights are enriched by a heavy dose of "psychodynamic" discourse.

My interpretation of this article is that it deals with aspects of socialization that have been dealt with many times. This effort to explain rather ordinary experiences in the lives of ten blind people was not improved, in my opinion, by the phenomenological and psychological vocabulary.

In Rowland's analysis, blind people are necessarily dependent on others, and in being so, give up their own dignity. I argue that most sighted people are dependent on others as well, from birth to death. It is a normal part of being human to experience periods of dependence. Just because a person continually seeks assistance in shopping and transportation (as in Rowland's examples) does not mean that essential values are lost in relationships. Symbiotic relationships frequently develop in which each contributes to the other, and dependency is not the issue for either. I have observed cases such as Rowland describes, in which one of a couple is frequently in the servant role and equal exchange is not apparent. However, I have also observed examples of mutual exchange, mutual benefit, and the absence of the feelings Mr. Rowland describes. All in all, my observations do not suggest that dependence is inherent in the condition of blindness.

BLINDNESS EMBEDDED IN CULTURE

Everything we know and say about blindness, we have learned from others in the culture and society in which we live. We may remember jokes or often repeated vignettes such as that of the four blind men feeling an elephant and not getting a complete picture. We acquire definitions from medical doctors and from social and behavioral scientists who study blind people. We also accumulate ideas and images from service providers, educators, and our mass media. In all cases, what we learn is related to other aspects of our culture: for example, beliefs about blindness relate to the employment and career interests of service providers and researchers who study blindness. Images about blindness do not randomly appear. Even in the folk culture of ordinary people, handed down ideas provide locally acceptable explanations about the origin of blindness or the proper status relationship between the sighted and the nonsighted.

To sociologists and anthropologists, culture usually refers to the generally shared outlook on life and characterizes ways people respond to situations. Societies, institutions, tools, techniques for solving problems, norms of appropriate behavior, and emotional attitudes are all interrelated in a given culture. They are perpetuated by enduring social structures, those institutions that formalize arrangements for socializing the next generation: the family, the school, religion, and so on. From a heightened awareness of one's culture, a person can approximate an understanding of how most individuals think, feel, or relate to events or others they happen to encounter.

A heightened awareness of other cultural arrangements can also arise from living in or studying other cultures. One soon realizes that blindness is regarded in many different ways around the world. Likewise, we gain insight by knowing how the conditions experienced by blind people have changed over time in any given society. For example, blind people in Spain live in very different economic circumstances today than they did before an organization of blind people, the Organización Nacional de Ciegos Españoles (ONCE), obtained government permission in 1938 to run as a business the largest national lottery in Spain. Now more than 40,000 people have a lucrative source of employment that was not available to them before the ONCE was created. Hence, Mr. Rowland's middle class examples present a limited and incomplete picture. His work reflects the predominate cultural arrangements, but he forgot that many people, such as the poor in rural areas, do not share equally in the arrangement thought necessary for a "good life." To be fair to Mr. Rowland, several of his more recent publications reflect a broader perspective than the one presented in his book, *Being-Blind-In-The-World.* I have included some of his important published writings in Chapter 5 dealing with sub-Saharan Africa.

In addition, every culture has undercurrents. There are frequently groups of people who, while sharing in many values of their culture, work to change some conditions which are judged harmful. They have not rejected the culture, but are merely trying to change certain features of it. For example, in the United States, we often hear the slogan: "We are changing what it means to be blind."

A society and its culture is made up of interacting individuals. Each person lives in what has been called "life space," which evolves from each person's accumulated experience in previous years. These individuals often relate to others in recurring ways, such as in families and in interest groups with shared goals. The results are social movements and organizations with identifiable patterns of interaction and ways of solving problems. Patterns of these enduring arrangements are often described as cultural values or cultural traits. There is nothing mysterious about these general concepts, just as there is nothing mysterious about blindness. Ideas about blindness change as a result of the activities of blind individuals, their interaction with others, and the eventual education of less well informed people in the same culture. As we will see in the next chapter, scientists and professionals are major creators of ideas about blindness in most affluent, industrial societies. But to illustrate a different perspective in a setting perhaps unfamiliar to most readers of this book, I will briefly review aspects of a subculture of blind people living in a Mexican village.

BLINDNESS IN A MEXICAN VILLAGE

We easily take for granted ideas we have about blindness and the social arrangements we have created to handle or manage blind people. Mr. Rowland's examples, previously discussed, illustrate the "experience of blindness" primarily in middle class family settings in a relatively prosperous, industrialized society, yet he concluded that he was describing aspects of blindness as a unique human experience. However, the "experience of blindness" differs greatly in Gwaltney's (1970) ethnographic description of blind people and their relations with others in a poor, remote Mexican village. The village of San Pedro Yolox had fewer than 1,000 inhabitants when Gwaltney studied it, and was almost entirely comprised of people with a distinct Indian heritage.

Residents in this village did not have a scientific, medical explanation for why blindness occurred. The most common explanation was that it was punishment from God. For example, a man who stole from the church and used the money to get drunk became blind as a punishment from God. When vision began to fail and his eyes were "finally closed" the situation was explained in terms of the man's "bad faith" (p. 101). "The blinding sickness was never attributed to sorcery. Expressions like, 'God closed his eyes completely,' 'God clouded his eyes' and 'God ended his sight' in common usage among the villagers, indicate a common tendency to ascribe blindness to supernatural intervention" (p. 103).

This village experienced a relatively high incidence of blindness. Almost all cases were diagnosed as onchocerciasis. Men more frequently incurred this disease, possibly because they often worked out of doors while not wearing shirts, which made them easier targets for the fly that helps spread the parasite. The infectious agent is the worm "onchocerca vovulus," which is transmitted by the intermediate host, a black fly of the genus "simulium." "Progressive lodging of the microfilanae of ochocerea voluls in the optic humors, the cornea, the iris and the sheath of the optic nerve may lead to acute visual impairment and even total blindness" (p. 191). The local villagers had no folk knowledge of this source of adult onset blindness in their village.

For the villagers, the most serious consequence of blindness was the inability to do labor. Begging became an activity of all the blind residents of this village, not only locally, but in preferred nearby towns as well. Although most sighted residents preferred that begging occur outside San Pedro Yolox, some begging did take place in the village in distinct forms: "village bounty consists almost exclusively of small donations of food. A beggar is either invited to share a meal or a few tortillas are placed in the basket which is carried to receive such donations" (p. 112).

Mobility in the rough, broken terrain of this village was not easy for anyone, much less for blind people. Because of the difficulty of travel, blind people in this village relied almost exclusively on "child guides."

"One of the major social consequences of onchocerciasis has been the amplification of the relationship between two groups at either extremity of the life course. The role of Lazaro is well established among village children. Adults act more rarely as guides but villagers look upon the service as being mutually beneficial and especially appropriate when rendered by young children" (p. 113).

Children led the blind by the hand and everyone viewed this as "natural." The children guided blind people on begging expeditions to other villages and accompanied them at village fiestas. Children learned their procedure by watching older children perform guide services. "Children do not call themselves guides nor do they generally refer to their services as guiding. A game of marbles, a storytelling session, an impromptu street interview was frequently prematurely but politely broken off as one or more of my younger friends and informants dashed off to 'walk' with one of the village blind persons" (p. 113). To the villagers, it would have been folly for blind people to try to travel alone on the rough terrain of the village and its environs. In San Pedro Yolox there were no special institutions or public arrangements to assist blind people. There was, however, empathy for those unfortunate enough to be blind. The child guides were an informal response to what the villagers saw as the obvious need of blind people for travel assistance. "Though blind and sighted villagers make guarded private accusations of undue parsimony and excessive mendicancy, no sighted Yoleno ever complained about the demands of their blind paisanos upon their time and empathy" (p. 114).

Kindly treatment was thought appropriate for blind people because their fate could have been anyone's fate. Blind people were thought to be under the protection of God: snakes would not bite them, nor lightning strike them, nor steep chasms injure them. God had inspired a "natural desire" for villagers to help the blind and planted love in the hearts of children who were eager to be guides (p.111). According to Gwaltney, the prevailing belief that the parasitically-induced blindness is the consequence of omnipotent, arbitrary divine intervention tends toward the emergence of "an essentially accommodative cultural response" (pp. v-vi). Both poverty and blindness were ancient features of the cultural landscape of this village; both were associated with a fatalism linked to "God's will". There was also suspicion of outsiders trying to change the village, which included doubts about government efforts to eradicate the disease causing blindness.

Finally, it is obvious that the experience of blindness in this traditional Mexican village is totally different from that described by Mr. Rowland in South Africa. In the Mexican village, inter-generational relationships are based upon child guides and accommodative attitudes resulting from a commonly held religious belief system. In South Africa, relationships are established with educators and welfare workers who understand the source and problems of blindness in scientific terms.

The Social Context of Blindness

Each of us is born into a particular culture where we learn to share a way of life with those around us. Culture here includes all that we know and all the things we make, including social arrangements and organized activities. Each of us is unique because we are born into a particular culture at a particular place and time in which social relationships are ongoing. The present life we experience is made up of all our preceding historical/social moments and our reactions to these experiences.

The location or situation we occupy in a particular culture is also important. For example, whether or not we are born in a rural area or large city has implications for the kind of rehabilitation or education services available. Family economic resources also, in part, determine the range of opportunities available to a blind child or newly blinded adult. For example, it is doubtless significant that Hellen Keller was born into a prosperous family that could afford a private teacher. Sullivan had the benefit of being associated with the Perkins School for the Blind. In my own case, I was fortunate to have been born into a caring family and into a society which had developed programs that provided enough educational and rehabilitation services for those who required them.

In most cases our lives, regardless of where we live, are a series of social encounters. These frequently involve direct contact with others, but can be experienced in other ways, for example, vicariously through literature. In the next section, I will distinguish between recurring patterns of social interaction, between the process of socialization and the more enduring structures or institutions we encounter.

SOCIAL INTERACTION

Socialization refers to the life long social experience in which individuals develop their human potential and become accustomed to their particular culture. Each of us becomes human when we learn to use language and relate to others. When a person becomes blind, he or she is faced with new conditions which frequently result in altered relationships with others. The individual has much to learn and is suddenly confronted by parents, friends, teachers and service providers who may have widely different ideas about blindness and future prospects. Although it was written nearly thirty years ago, no one, at least in the English language, has significantly improved on Robert Scott's *The Making of Blind Men* (1969). Scott begins by discussing folk and psychological opinions about blindness in the United States. Folk opinions, supposedly based on "common sense," maintain that blind people experience unique versions of sadness, frustration, helplessness, and docility, and that playfulness and joking are out of character (p.4). On the other hand, psychologists hold that there are patterns to the behavior demonstrated by blind people as they deal with two conditions: "the psychological reactions that all blind people have to becoming blind and the enduring impact of the condition upon basic components of personality" (p. 6). Scott concludes that people who become blind experience grief and depression at first, but through the period of adjustment, they begin to display many different kinds of behavior.

What they display is, of course, derived from interaction with others. According to Scott, "The disability of blindness is a learned social role. The various attitudes and patterns of behavior that characterize people who are blind are not inherent in their condition but, rather, are acquired through the ordinary processes of social learning. Thus, there is nothing inherent in the condition of blindness that requires a person to be docile, dependent, melancholy or helpless" (p. 14). In addition, if we can acquire an understanding of a person's self image (the set of beliefs, feelings and attitudes he holds about himself), we can understand a great deal about him. For Scott, a person's identity or self concept is basic or "at the heart of" his experience as a "socialized human being" (p. 15). One's self image develops as one sees himself in relation to the expectations of others. "Because of this, the substance of a man's self image largely consists of his perceptions of the evaluations that others make of him, and particularly those others whose opinions he values most highly" (p.15). Thus, he learns that he is rewarded for behaving in ways others judge appropriate.

Socialization occurs in three main contexts: in early childhood, in face-to-face interaction with sighted people, and from the organizations created to help blind people (pp.16-17). Scott thinks that the importance of this third arena of socialization cannot be overemphasized. "Through this complicated network of organizations, agencies and programs for the blind, the phenomenon of blindness in our society has literally been transformed" (p.18). Involvement with blindness agencies results in three types of people:

> . . . those who have completed rehabilitation and vocational training and are now living independently in their home communities; those who have delib-

erately disengaged themselves from blindness organizations in order to make a living by begging and blinded veterans of the armed forces of the United States, most of whom receive special rehabilitation, medical and financial benefits because of their blindness. (pp.105-106)

According to Scott, the number of people who returned to their jobs or found competitive employment after encountering blindness agencies is, "in all probability, quite small" (p. 108). Scott labels as the "independent blind" those who have managed to avoid dependency relationships with agencies and who are involved in ordinary life in the community. He states that those who succeed are unusual; they have peculiar qualities not related to being blind. "While it is not a necessary condition for independence, blind people who manage to live independent lives often have either an independent income or some special and unusual quality or talent or both" (p. 108). In fairness, he does admit to basing his comments on interviews with only six blind people "in this category" (p. 109).

Professor Scott has described several important ingredients of the socialization process. He has shown quite convincingly the process by which blind people become dependent upon agencies. However, I have three criticisms of his approach. First, he leaves out or largely ignores the reflective aspect of self development. Individuals are more than the passive objects of socialization experiences. For humans, there is frequently a mental process which mediates between the stimuli received and the responses made. It is in this arena that we have the feeling of being self-determined, that within the array of alternatives available to us, we occasionally make self-conscious decisions. I suspect that blind people do this with the same frequency as anyone else.

Second, the variety of responses to agency and community socialization efforts is, based on my observations, more varied than Professor Scott's work suggests. Many blind people live independent lives who do not have an assured level of income and who do not have "some special and unusual quality or talent, or both" (p. 108). Writing only six years after the appearance of Scott's book, Lowenfeld voiced a similar criticism of Scott:

While the almost one hundred people may well represent the blind within the blindness system, the six cannot possibly have given him a clear appreciation of the beliefs, attitudes and adjustments of the hundreds of blind teachers, the hundreds of blind lawyers, the hundreds of computer experts and the hundreds of independent businessmen, to name only a few occupations in which we know hundreds of blind people to be engaged.(p. 291)

My third criticism of Professor Scott's work is his almost complete neglect of one extremely important source of reference group behavior for blind people: the experience of other blind people. In every society, individuals with similar interests act in consort, creating organizations to promote their collective interests. In the United States, for example, blind people have created large, nationwide organizations to promote equal opportunity for blind people and positive images about blindness. Many individual blind people, as this book illustrates, are often significantly influenced by exposure to positive role models: other blind people who have successfully solved the problems that each individual confronts. Organizations of the blind frequently have significant levels of organizational resources, money, staff and committed volunteers which are used to introduce newly blind people to more positive images and experiences of blindness. Nationwide organizations of blind people had existed for more than twenty-five years in the United States and had been significant in positive socialization experiences of many blind people when Scott wrote, facts that he did not specifically mention or barely alluded to in *The Making of Blind Men.*

During the period of Professor Scott's research and to a lesser degree, today, the largest organization of blind people in the United States has been in an adversarial relationship with many agencies. A researcher who focuses his attention on these agencies and the socialization of individuals may only be minimally exposed to the activities of consumer organizations. Many blind people themselves never encounter consumer organizations. Yet it is puzzling to me why there appears to be almost studied inattention to the potential these organizations represent for providing positive socialization experiences. For example, another social scientist who studied the importance of the self concept is Dean Tuttle in *Self-Esteem and Adjusting to Blindness: The Process of Responding to Life's Demands* (1984). Tuttle analyzes problems individuals have in adjusting to the "trauma of blindness." Using trauma either as a medical or psychological concept, he describes it as a severe condition requiring significant intervention and often having lasting consequences. Because blindness is so traumatic, professional help is usually required. Like Scott, Tuttle largely ignores consumer organizations and the important role other blind people may have in the developing self concept of a blind person. While discussing signif-icant others and reference groups, he advises that a blind person should be introduced to a teacher, school superintendent, counselor, or friend and at one point goes so far as to suggest that one meet another blind person to learn some practical strategies. "The profes-sional may want to arrange for a competent blind person to meet with the individual who is mourning. Areas of concern to be discussed with the recently blinded might include some 'tricks of the trade' or some quickly and easily learned adaptive techniques" (pp. 77-78). Based on my own experience, it would be more useful to be introduced to the wide array of educational materials produced by organizations of blind people and to more blind people who have solved many prob-lems in different ways.

ORGANIZED SERVICES

Organized responses to blindness vary from culture to culture. The extent of these organizations varies with the economic resources avail-able and the presence of cultural values that support public interven-tion to educate, rehabilitate, or in other ways take care of blind peo-ple. Without the necessary humanitarian value tradition, organizations for the blind may not develop. This was the case in China, described later in Chapter 5, where Western-style approaches to intervention came with the second wave of Christian missionaries, beginning short-ly after the Opium War with Britain in the 1840s.

Organizations which provide services to blind people are important for several reasons. In, *The Making of Blind Men,* Scott describes how they socialize blind people in the United States. The organizations and educational institutions, some of which I discuss in Chapter 3 and 4, are important because of their activity in the cultural production of new images about blindness. In some countries, they are important as they become the focus of conflict between themselves and consumer organizations. Although frequently intended to rehabilitate and edu-cate blind people for participation in wider society, they can become an actual barrier to normal participation. Because of fund raising appeals and public relation efforts, ordinary citizens may come to think of these agencies as the "place where you send blind people." The agencies are also important because they represent a significant economic resource potentially available to blind people. No one has been more articulate than Jacobus tenBroek, founder of the National Federation of the Blind, in describing the harmful features of agency behavior. In his article, "Within the Grace of God" (1956), he accused the agencies of assuming the roles of protectors and interpreters of the blind and of attributing to blind people characteristics of abnormality and dependency to justify agency practices.

Despite much consumer unrest and questions about the effectiveness of disability programs, little attention has been paid to the organizational context in which rehabilitation services occur. Scott discussed several ways organizations served the blind, including the screening of clients to best serve their needs and the process by which economic goals gradually replace earlier goals of rehabilitation or education (Scott 1967). But because there was more to say, I have stressed the work setting of agency personnel and their support systems: professional organizations and graduate training programs (Vaughan, 1993). Although Albrecht (1992) had studied the economic aspects of the rehabilitation system as a whole, I emphasized patterns of domination within bureaucracies and between bureaucratically organized agencies and their clients.

Max Weber linked the growth of bureaucratic structure to the control of economic resources, which he thought to be central to the creation of wealth and power. "The bureaucratic structure goes hand in hand with the concentration of material means of management in the hands of the master" (p. 980). Weber noted that bureaucratic structures pervade all areas of society, and that they may be based on custom or tradition or more recent norms of efficiency. Although bureaucratic organizations and styles of management vary from culture to culture, they all have at least one feature in common: a pattern of domination and subordination. Regarding organizations created to provide services to blind people, these organizations frequently became the only economic resources available, leaving blind people few options.

In extending his analysis to the modern welfare state, Weber found that patterns of economic influence and the degree of political domination vary with the size of the activity in question. Holders of political and economic resources, including cultural transmission institutions, are the focus of our efforts to understand persistently enduring structures of relationships which alter the life chances of subordinate groups.

For a blind person, the rehabilitation process usually begins with a physician who determines the applicant's eligibility for services. Following referral to an agency, the applicant will usually be one of a larger number of people participating in the rehabilitation program at the same time. Different professionals evaluate various aspects of the client, including intelligence, level of social adjustment, mobility skills, personal grooming, vocational interests, and so on. In this context, blind consumers can be viewed as commodities or the raw materials from which end products are to be produced. Throughout the program, these people are cases to be processed by the various workers involved. The client may spend many hours doing nothing while awaiting events scheduled for the convenience of the organization. Procedures regarded as ordinary by the organization may appear to the client as silly, unnecessary, demeaning, arbitrary, and seemingly endless. "The client feels himself or herself continually being considered as a type or category of a problem rather than as a whole person. The notion of 'red tape' is used universally to describe the frustration ordinary citizens feel in dealing with bureaucratic requirements, and there is a full measure of it here" (Vaughan, 1993, p. 51).

In a setting fraught with anxiety, where the client feels powerless and without alternatives, organizational procedures can be experienced as extremely burdensome and demoralizing. Scott noted that counselors often define blindness as a severe problem requiring long-term intervention. "Discrediting the client's personal ideas about his problem is achieved in several ways. His initial statements about why he has come to the organization and what he hopes to receive from it are euphemistically termed 'the presenting problem,' a phrase that implies superficiality in the client's view" (Scott, 1969, p. 77). Long-term involvement in the agency's program may be prescribed. If the client seriously questions the recommended procedures, maladjustment may be the diagnosis. Deference and compliance are presumed: the demeanor due to those of superior knowledge and training (Larson, 1977, p. 157).

Clients are processed in a wide array of settings, most of which have similar organizational characteristics. These include schools for the blind, sheltered workshops, special program centers (usually called

"associations for the blind" or "lighthouses"), and residential rehabilitation centers. In addition, in the United States, there are federal and
state vocational rehabilitation programs and large privately funded
national programs such as the American Foundation for the Blind.
Those special places are locally well known because of their fund raising appeals and public relations efforts. All industrialized societies, to
some extent, have organizations similar to those just mentioned in the
United States. In Chapter 7, I describe the opposite situation where, in
Spain, the ONCE, an organization owned and controlled by blind
people themselves provides, nationwide, education and rehabilitation
services. There are also many large international organizations, some
of which were founded in the age of colonialism and frequently associated with religious organizations. For example, these are Sight
Savers International, Helen Keller International, and Christoffel
Blindenmission, to mention only a few. Regardless of the size or the
extent of geographic concern, these agencies demonstrate similar patterns of bureaucratic organization.

In *Professions and Power*, Johnson (1967) noted that the political
dimensions of professions do not always reflect disembodied societal
needs. Social welfare and educational activities alike differentiate
power in relationships among the participants. As representatives of
the organized structure of power, social services personnel are
employees dependent upon the ongoing processes of the organization
for their livelihood. There are few employment alternatives except at
similar highly specialized bureaucratic agencies. Consequently, there
is pressure, as Weber noted, for personnel to become extensions of the
inherent power arrangements (Vaughan, 1993). This condition results
in defense of vested interests. The social control and domination of
subordinates, work specialization supported by claims to expertise,
and a refined and developed rhetoric justify the entire process. Thus,
a culturally created social arrangement (the rationally organized
bureaucracy) leads to a somewhat similar pattern of service delivery in
all industrialized nations and international organizations are now
extending it into less economically developed regions of the world.
Except for the research of Roberto Garvía on the ONCE (see Chapter
7), I am not yet aware of research that would answer the question of
whether or not a large bureaucratically-arranged organization owned
by blind people themselves is able to avoid the harmful consequences
of domination.

BLINDNESS AND THE NEW WORLD ORDER

Shortly after World War I, the International Labor Organization (ILO) was created to promote improved conditions for laborers in all countries. Near the end of World War II, the Western allies agreed on general strategies for rebuilding economies devastated by the war. The United Nations soon arose as the major arena for promoting international cooperation. Subsequently, additional international governmental organizations were created such as the World Health Organization (WHO) and the International Monetary Fund (IMF). In his 1991 State of the Union Address following the Gulf War with Iraq, President George Bush spoke of international cooperation to help bring about a "New World Order." At first glance, it may seem farfetched, but rehabilitation programs are being standardized through the influence of these organizations, particularly through agencies related to the United Nations and the ILO. In fact, I have observed some of these developments while participating in international conferences regarding rehabilitation in the People's Republic of China (1991), the United Nations in New York (1994), Thailand (1994), Ghana (1996), and Spain (1997).

For example, I participated in the First Africa Forum on Rehabilitation held in Accra, Ghana, April 22-26, 1996. The leaders of organizations of blind people from eleven different African nations participated as well as representatives from several different international nongovernment organizations (NGOs). Consultants also represented the UN, ILO, and WHO. I was very impressed by the quality of leadership displayed by organizations of blind people from these various countries. In many cases, organizational and leadership development has been encouraged by economic resources and consultants provided by the NGOs. This first Africa Forum was under the able leadership of Mr. Aubrey Webson of the Hilton-Perkins International Program.

Almost all developing countries focus attention on economic development at the expense of social development, including rehabilitation services. For several decades, international government organizations have been a major external funding service. International organizations such as the UN and the ILO have insisted that rehabilitation services be general in scope and community-based. Generalized rehabilitation services have traditionally been opposed by the organized blind and professionals who provide education and rehabilitation services to blind people. I view the issue of generalized services from the experience of the organized blind movement in the United States. In the nineteenth century, people assumed that asylums were an improvement because they separated blind people from the mentally ill, physically malformed, and economically impoverished. In addition, schools to educate blind people also developed in the United States in the nineteenth century and much was learned from them. Subsequently, many professionals and blind people have developed "mainstreaming," now sometimes called "full inclusion" (see Chapter 4).

At first glance these developments seem auspicious. It was surely desirable for blind students to be educated in the same schools and social environments as their sighted peers. However, in the past decade many articles have appeared which raise questions about the consequences of "mainstreaming" and "full inclusion" for blind students. In general, regular teachers and even special education teachers are seldom prepared to teach the unique skills required by blind students such as Braille, mobility skills, and other skills for independent living. "The present difficulty is yet one more manifestation of the same old problem in a field in which there are many different disabilities and which even students with the same deficit have very different needs; no one educational solution will ever fit everybody" (Pierce, 1994, p. 71).

The issue of students being placed in an institution or a community is not the basic problem, according to Fred Schroeder in his 1994 *Monitor* article, "Expectations: The Critical Factor in the Education of Blind Children." Even if special education teachers are technically proficient in meeting the needs of blind children, something more basic must be present. "What is needed, therefore, is not the refinement or fine tuning of this system or that. Instead, all systems must be premised on a fundamental belief in the ability of blind children to compete—each system must begin with this belief and translate it into expectations" (Schroeder, 1994, p. 102). This belief includes the understanding that blind children are inherently normal, as much as other children are normal, and can compete in most areas if taught by competent teachers with positive attitudes about blindness.

Many parents of blind children, and blind people in general, are concerned about what may be lost in "full inclusion" types of programs. Despite possible social benefits, illiteracy among blind people in the United States has been on the rise. Whether it be a single blind child in a larger class or one or two blind children in separate special classes intended to teach skills to disabled children, most do not learn basic communication and travel skills as well as they might in schools that specialize in the education of blind children.

In this light, I have viewed the trend toward generalized rehabilitation services being recommended for less economically developed countries. When resources are scarce, specialized schools for blind children are too expensive. The least costly approach is to provide generalized rehabilitation services based in the local community. For example, the International Labor Organization recommends that "emphasis must be on providing services: for all categories of disability, for equality of opportunities, for facilitating access to mainstream services and careers, and for involving disabled people, through their organizations at every stage of development" (*Towards Equalizing Opportunities,* 1994, p. 5). Hence, countries are encourage to design rehabilitation services to meet the needs of all disabled people. Likewise, workers must "cross train" in order to work in any area of rehabilitation and even in the more general field of placement for unemployed people, whether or not they have disabilities (*International Labor Standards,* 1984). Community-based rehabilitation programs occur in the setting of general economic development programs. People with disabilities are directed to utilize volunteers and any type of locally available rehabilitation resources, while existing programs should change to meet the "new policy" concerning comprehensive, community-based services.   "Nongovernment Organizations (NGOs), their services and institutions would have to conform to the new policy of a country, particularly if the voluntary sector is to be a major service provider in the future" (ILO, p. 9). In addition, government officials and offices are ordered to monitor the quality of programs provided by private agencies (NGOs).

Large, well-established international organizations such as the UN and ILO have considerable prestige and influence in many parts of the world. In the past, they have represented economic resources or have been major players in a network of organizations that control a significant percentage of funds for development programs. The UN, ILO, and WHO influence the thinking of government officials who have responsibility for developing economic and education programs in each country. Frequently, these government officials know little about rehabilitation and much less about blindness rehabilitation. They have more incentive to cooperate with international organizations that represent external funding than to listen to organizations of blind people within their own countries. Many of the organizations of blind people are relatively new and have not yet developed the political clout necessary to combat the influence of these international organizations. It is extremely important that blind people in developing countries continue to develop strong leadership and strong organizations. They and some private nongovernment organizations may be the only advocates for programs to enable blind people to live independently.

Mindful that every culture is different, I am confident that blind people can live independently and participate fully in society anywhere they live. One participant in the first Africa Forum, a well-educated and successful blind person, told me that if community-based rehabilitation had been the only thing available, he would likely now be involved in basket weaving in a small village. Basket weaving may be a desirable occupation, but blind people should not be confined solely to this type of employment.

POLITICAL CONTEXT

National policies related to disability programs may expand or contract with the economic or political fortunes of a given society. In Chapter 5, I illustrate how programs for disabled people, including blind people, changed dramatically with the revolution led by Mao Tsi-Tung and the Chinese Communist Party. An especially dramatic change in the life situation of many blind people came about from the economic reforms which led to the free market economy under the leadership of Dong Xioping. In my earlier book, I described the increase in the categories of disability and the increase in the number of people receiving disability benefits. In the United States, the decade of the 1980s (Matras, 1990, p. 270) also saw a dramatic increase in the number of people receiving disability benefits. Whatever caused this increase is in the economic interest of the rehabilitation industry. It also may be politically desirable to remove large numbers of people from the labor force; unemployment rates are lower than they otherwise might be. Disability rates may change as the occupational structure changes (Nagi, 1981, p. 41).

When economic resources are scarce, political decisions are made concerning which kinds of physical conditions require public intervention. In Poland, for example, impairment, disability and handicap are not perceived as pertinent issues because there are more urgent problems that have to be settled, such as the prevalence of acute communicable diseases or high infant mortality rates (Sokolowska et al.). These authors describe the political process by which government funding is made available to make rehabilitation services and occupation opportunities available as the Polish economy expands (23).

Blind people themselves sometimes create large organizations, become active in the political process, and address issues of interest to blind people themselves. They usually focus on unfair social conditions and unequal social relationships. "It is an unadaptive, unhelpful environment which needs to be examined and changed. Being interested in disabled people requires an examination of those material conditions and social relations which contribute to their dehumanization and isolation" (Baxter, p. 5).

IS BLINDNESS SIMPLY A CHARACTERISTIC?

We have already observed that blindness occurs in every culture, and that blindness itself does not create any particular social arrangements. According to one view, a view which I endorse, blindness is simply and only a characteristic of individuals. No one has made this argument more strongly than Dr. Kenneth Jernigan, President of the North American Caribbean Region of the World Blind Union and President Emeritus of the National Foundation of the Blind of the United States. The following is a condensed version of his article, "Blindness: Handicap or Characteristic?" published in the July 1996 issues of the World Blind.

Blindness: Handicap or Characteristic?

One prominent authority in the rehabilitation of blind people recently said, "Loss of sight is dying. When, in the full current of his sighted life, blindness comes on a man, it is the end, the death, of that sighted life . . . It is superficial, if not naive, to think of blindness as a blow to the eyes only, to sight only. It is a destructive blow to the self-image of a man . . . a blow almost to his being itself!"

This is one view, a view held by a substantial number of people in the world today. But it is not the only view. In my opinion it is not the correct view. What is blindness? Is it a "dying"?

A Characteristic

No one is likely to disagree with me if I say that blindness, first of all, is a characteristic. But a great many people will disagree when I go on to say that blindness is only a characteristic. It is nothing more or less than that. It is nothing more special, more peculiar or more terrible than that suggests. When we understand the nature of blindness as a characteristic—a normal characteristic like hundreds of others with which each of us must live—we shall better understand the real needs to be met by agencies serving the blind, as well as the false needs which should not be met.

By definition, a characteristic—any characteristic—is a limitation. A white house, for example, is a limited house; it cannot be green or blue or red; it is limited to being white. Likewise every characteristic—those we regard as strengths as well as those we regard as weaknesses—is a limitation. Each one forces us to some extent into a mold: each restricts to some degree the range of possibility, of flexibility and very often of opportunity as well. Blindness is such a limitation. Are blind people more limited than others?

Take a sighted person with an average mind (something not too hard to locate); take a blind person with a superior mind (something not impossible to locate) – and then make all the other characteristics of these two exactly equal (something which certainly is impossible). Now, which of the two is more limited? It depends, of course, on what you want them to do. If you are choosing up sides for baseball, then the blind person is more limited– that is, he or she is "handicapped." If you are hunting somebody to teach history or to figure out your income tax, the sighted person is more limited or "handicapped."

Many human characteristics are obvious limitations; others are not so obvious. Poverty (the lack of material means, is one of the most obvious. Ignorance (the lack of knowledge or education) is another. Old age (the lack of youth and vigor) is yet another. Blindness (the lack of eyesight) is still another. In all these cases the limitations are apparent or seem to be. But let us look at some other common characteristics which do not seem limiting. Take the very opposite of old age—youth. Is age a limitation in the case of a youth of twenty? Indeed it is, for a person who is twenty will not be considered for most responsible positions, especially supervisory or leadership positions. He or she may be entirely mature, fully capable, in every way qualified for the job. Even so, age will bar the person from employment. He or she will be classified as too green and immature to handle the responsibility. And even if the person were to land the position, others on the job would almost certainly resent being supervised by so young. The characteristic of being twenty is definitely a limitation.

The same holds true for any other age. Take age fifty, which many regard as the prime of life. The person of fifty does not have the physical vigor he or she had at twenty; and, indeed, most companies (despite recent legislation to the contrary) will not start a new employee at that age. When I first wrote those words in the 1960s, the Bell Telephone System (yes, it was the Bell System at that time) had a general prohibition against hiring anybody over the age of thirty-five. But it is interesting to note that the United States Constitution has a prohibition against having anybody under thirty-five run for President. The moral is plain: any age carries its built-in limitations.

Let us take another unlikely handicap—not that of ignorance, but its exact opposite. Can it be said that education is ever a handicap? The answer is definitely yes. In the agency which I headed (I was Director of the Iowa Commission for the Blind from 1958 to 1978), I would not have hired Albert Einstein under any circumstances if he had been alive and available. His fame (other people would have continually flocked to the agency and prevented us from doing our work) and his intelligence (he would have been bored to madness by the routine of most of our jobs) would both have been too severe as limitations.

Here is an actual case in point. When I was Director of the Iowa Commission for the Blind, a vacancy occurred on the library staff. Someone was needed to perform certain clerical duties and take charge of shelving and checking books. After all applicants had been screened, the final choice came down to two. Applicant A had a college degree, was seemingly alert, and clearly had more than average intelligence. Applicant B had a high school diploma (no college), and was of average intelligence and possessed only moderate initiative. I hired Applicant B. Why? Because I suspected that Applicant A would regard the work as beneath him, would soon become bored with its undemanding assignments, and would leave as soon as something better came along. I would then have to find and train another employee. On the other hand, I felt that Applicant B would consider the work interesting and even challenging, that he was thoroughly capable of handling the job, and that he would be not only an excellent but also a permanent employee. In fact, he worked out extremely well.

In other words, in that situation the characteristic of education—the possession of a college degree—was a limitation and a handicap. Even above-average intelligence was a limitation, and so was a high level of initiative. There is a familiar bureaucratic label for this unusual disadvantage: it is the term "overqualified."

A Limitation

This should be enough to make the point—which is that if blindness is a limitation (and, indeed, it is), it is so in quite the same way as innumerable other characteristics to which human flesh is heir. I believe that blindness has no more importance than any of a hundred other characteristics and that the average blind person is able to perform the average job in the average place of business, and do it as effectively as the average sighted person similarly situated. The above average can compete with the above average, the average with the average, and the below average with the below average—provided (and it is a large proviso) that he or she is given training and opportunity.

Often when I have advanced this proposition, I have been met with the response, "But you can't look at it that way. Just consider what you might have done if you had been sighted and still had all the other capacities you now possess."

"Not so," I reply. "We do not compete against what we might have been, but only against other people as they now are, with their combination of strengths and weaknesses, handicaps and limitations." If we are going down that track, why not ask me what I might have done if I had been born with Rockefeller's money, the brains of Einstein, the physique of the young Joe Louis and the persuasive abilities of Franklin Roosevelt? (And do I need to remind anyone, in passing, that FDR was severely handicapped physically?) I wonder if anyone ever said to him: "Mr President, just consider what you might have done if you had not had polio!"

Others have said to me, "But I formerly had sight, so I know what I am missing." To which I might reply, "And I was formerly twenty, so I know what I am missing." Does this mean that I should spend my time grieving for the past? Or alternatively should I deal with my current situation, sizing up its possibilities and problems and turning them to my advantage? Our characteristics are constantly changing, and we are forever acquiring new experiences, limitations and assets. We do not compete against what we formerly were but against other people as they now are.

In a recent magazine article, a blinded veteran, who is now a college professor, puts forward a notion of blindness radically different from this. He sets the limitations of blindness apart from all others and makes them unique. Having done this, he can say that all other human characteristics, strengths and weaknesses belong in one category—and that with regard to them the blind and the sighted are just about equal. But the blind person also has the additional and unique limitation of blindness. Therefore, there is really nothing the blind person can do quite as well as the sighted person, and he or she can continue to hold his or her job only because there are charity and goodness in the world.

What this blind professor does not observe is that the same distinction he makes regarding blindness can be made with equal plausibility with respect to any of a dozen—perhaps a hundred—of other characteristics. For example, suppose we distinguish intelligence from all other traits as uniquely different. Then the person with above 125 IQ is just about the same as the person with below

125 IQ–except for intelligence. Therefore, the college professor with less than 125 IQ cannot really do anything as well as the person with more than 125 IQ –and can continue to hold his or her job only because there are charity and goodness in the world.

"Are we going to assume," says this blind professor, "that all blind people are so wonderful in all other areas that they easily make up for any limitations imposed by loss of sight? I think not." But why, I ask, should we single out the particular characteristic of blindness? We might just as well specify some other. For instance, are we going to assume that all people with less than 125 IQ are so wonderful in all others that they easily make up for any limitations imposed by lack of intelligence? I think not.

A Handicap

This consideration brings us to the problem of terminology and semantics– and therewith to the heart of the matter of blindness as a handicap. The assumption that the limitation of blindness is so much more severe than others that it warrants being singled out for special definition is built into the very warp and woof of our language and psychology.

Blindness conjures up a condition of unrelieved disaster -- something much more terrible and dramatic than other limitations. Moreover, blindness is a conspicuously visible limitation, and there are not so many blind people around that there is any danger that the rest of the population will become accustomed to it or take it for granted. If all of those in our midst who possess an IQ under 125 exhibited, say, green stripes on their faces, I suspect that they would begin to be regarded as inferior to the non-striped–and that there would be immediate and tremendous discrimination.

When someone says to a blind person, "You do things so well that I forget you are blind–I simply think of you as being like anybody else," is that really a compliment? Suppose one of us went to France, and someone said: "You do things so well that I forget you are an American and simply think of you as being like anyone else." Would it be a compliment? Of course, the blind person should not wear a chip on the shoulder or allow himself or herself to become angry or emotionally upset. The blind person should be courteous and should accept the statement as the compliment it is meant to be. But the blind person should also understand that it is really not complimentary. In reality it says: "It is normal for blind people to be inferior and limited, different and much less able than the rest of us. Of course, you are still a blind person and still much more limited than I, but you have compensated for it so well that I almost forget that you are my inferior."

The social attitudes about blindness are all-pervasive. Not only do they affect the sighted by the blind as well. This is one of the most troublesome problems which we have to face. Public attitudes about the blind too often become the attitudes of the blind. The blind tend to see themselves as others see them. They too often accept the public view of their limitations and thus do much to make those limitations a reality.

Several years ago, Dr. Jacob Freid (at that time a young teacher of sociology and later head of the Jewish Braille Institute of America) performed an interesting experiment. He gave a test in photograph identification to black and white students at the university where he was teaching. There was one photograph of a black woman in a living room of a home of culture—well furnished with paintings, sculpture, books and flowers. Asked to identify the person in the photograph, the students said she was a "cleaning woman," "housekeeper," "cook," "laundress," "servant," "domestic," or "nanny." The revealing insight is that the black students made the same identification as the white students. The woman was Mary McLeod Bethune, one of the most famous black women of her time, founder and president of Bethune-Cookman College, who held a top post during Franklin Roosevelt's administration and a person of brilliance and prestige in the world of higher education. What this incident tells us is that education, like nature, abhors a vacuum, and that when members of a minority group do not have correct and complete information about themselves, they accept the stereotypes of the majority group even when they are false and unjust. Even today, after so many years of the civil rights movement, one wonders how many blacks would make the traditional and stereotyped identification of the photograph—if not verbally, at least in their hearts.

Similarly with the blind—the public image is everywhere dominant. This is the explanation for the attitude of those blind persons who are ashamed to carry a white cane or who try to bluff sight which they do not possess. Although great progress is now being made, there are still many people (sighted as well as blind) who believe that blindness is not altogether respectable.

Alternatives

The blind person must devise alternative techniques to do many things which would be done with sight if he or she had normal vision. It will be observed that I say alternative, not substitute techniques, for the word "substitute" connotes inferiority, and the alternative techniques employed by the blind person need not be inferior to visual techniques. In fact, some are superior. Of course, some are inferior and some are equal.

In this connection it is interesting to consider the matter of flying. In comparison with the birds, humans begin at a disadvantage. They cannot fly. They have no wings. They are "handicapped." But humans see birds flying, and they long to do likewise. Humans cannot use the "normal," bird-like method, so they begin to devise alternative techniques. In jet airplanes humans now fly higher, father and faster than any bird that has ever existed. If humans had possessed wings, the airplane would probably never have been devised and the inferior wing-flapping method would still be in general use.

This matter of our irrational images and stereotypes with regard to blindness was brought sharply home to me in the early 1960s during the course of a rehabilitation conference in Little Rock, Arkansas. I found myself engaged in a discussion with Father Carroll, a well-known leader in the field of work with the blind at that time. Father Carroll held quite different views from those I have been advancing. The error in my argument about blindness as a characteristic, he advised me, was the blindness is not in the range of "normal" characteristics. Therefore, its limitations are radically different from those of other characteristics falling within the normal range. If a normal characteristic is simply one possessed by the majority in a group, then it is not normal to have a black skin in America or a white skin in the world at large. It is not normal to have red hair or to be over six feet tall. If, on the other hand, a normal characteristic is simply what this or some other authority defines as being normal, then we have a circular argument—one that gets us nowhere.

In this same discussion I put forward the theory that a person who was sighted and of average means and who had all other characteristics in common with a blind person of considerable wealth would be less mobile than the blind person. I had been arguing that there were alternative techniques (not substitute) for doing those things which one would do with sight if one had normal vision. Father Carroll, as well as several others, had been contending that there was no real, adequate substitute for sight in traveling about. I told the story of a wealthy blind person I know who goes to Hawaii or some other place every year and who hires sighted attendants and is much more mobile than any sighted person I know who has ordinary means since most of the people I know can't go to Hawaii at all. After all of the discussion and the fact that I thought I had conveyed some understanding of what I was saying, a participant in the conference said—as if he thought he was making a telling point—"Wouldn't you admit that the wealthy man in question would be even more mobile if he had his sight?"

Services for Blind People

This brings us to be subject of services to the blind, and more exactly to their proper scope and direction. There are, as I see it, four basic types of services now being provided to blind persons by public and private agencies and volunteer groups in this country. They are:

1. services based on the theory that blindness is uniquely different from other characteristics and that it carries with it permanent inferiority and severe limitations upon activity;

2. services aimed at teaching the blind person a new and constructive set of attitudes about blindness—based on the premise that the prevailing social attitudes, assimilated involuntarily by the blind person, are mistaken in content and destructive in effect;

3. services aimed at teaching alternative techniques and skills related to blindness; and

4. services not specifically related to blindness but to other characteristics (such as old age and lack of education), which are nevertheless labeled as "services to the blind."

For purposes of this discussion, categories three and four are not relevant since they are not central to the philosophical point at issue. We are concerned here with categories one and two. An illustration of the assumptions underlying the first of these four types of services (category one) is the statement quoted earlier which begins, "Loss of sight is dying." Father Carroll (who was the one who made the statement) elaborated on that tragic metaphor by pointing out that "the eye is a sexual symbol" and that, accordingly the man who has not eyes is not a "whole man." He cited the play Oedipus Rex as proof of his contention that the eye is a sexual symbol. I believe that this misses the whole point of the classic tragedy. Like many moderns, the Greeks considered the severest possible punishment to be the loss of sight. Oedipus committed a mortal sin. Unknowingly he had killed his father and married his mother. Therefore, his punishment must be correspondingly great. But that is just what his self-imposed blindness—a punishment, not a sexual symbol.

But Father Carroll's view not only misses the point of Oedipus Rex—it misses the point of blindness. And in so doing it misses the point of blindness and of services intended to aid the blind is mistaken. For according to this view, what the blind person needs most desperately is the help of a psychiatrist—of the kind so prominently in evidence at several of the centers and agencies for the blind throughout the United States. According to this view what the blind person needs most is not travel training but therapy. Blind persons will be taught to accept their limitations as insurmountable and their difference from others as unbridgeable. They will be encouraged to adjust to their painful station as second-class citizens and discouraged from any thought of breaking and entering the first-class compartment. Moreover, all of this will be done in the name of teaching them "independence" and a "realistic" approach to their blindness.

Resignation and Rebellion

The two competing types of services for the blind—categories one and two on my list of four—with their underlying conflict of philosophy may perhaps be clarified by a rather fanciful analogy. All of us recall the case of the Jews in Nazi Germany. Suddenly, in the 1930s, the German Jews were told by their society that they were "handicapped" person—that they were inferior to other Germans simply by virtue of being Jews. Given this social fact, what sort of adjustment services might we have offered to the victim of Jewishness? I suggest that there are two alternatives—matching categories one and two above.

First, since the Jews have been "normal" individuals until quite recently, it will, of course, be quite a shock (or "trauma" as modern lingo has it) for them to learn that they are permanently and constitutionally inferior to others and can engage only in a limited range of activities. They will, therefore require a psychiatrist to give them counseling and therapy and to reconcile them to their lot. They must "adjust" to their handicap and "learn to live" with the fact that they are not "whole men and women." If they are, as the propaganda would have it, "realistic," they may even manage to be happy. They can be taken to an adjustment center, where they may engage in a variety of routine activities suitable to Jews. Again, it should be noted that all of this will be done in the name of teaching them how to accept reality as Jews. This is one form of adjustment training.

In the case of Nazi Germany, of course, the so-called "adjustment training" for the Jews passed the bounds of sanity and ended in the death camps of the Holocaust. The custody and control with which we as blind persons deal do not generally in present-day society express themselves in such barbarous forms, but it should be remembered that blind babies were uniformly exposed on the hillsides to die in earlier times. Today's custodial attitudes about the blind are more often than not kindly meant—especially if the blind are submissive and grateful and if they are willing to stay in their place. In fact, with respect to the blind, the day of custodialism is hopefully passing.

We know what happened to the Jews and others in Nazi Germany who rejected the premise that Jewishness equalled inferiority. The problem was not in Jewishness but in the perceptions of others. Any real so-called "adjustment" would have needed to involve equal treatment and human rights. The problem was centered not in the individual but in society and society's perception of the individual. In such circumstances the psychiatrist (even if anybody had been inclined to use one) would not have been helpful.

The so-called professionalism of the Nazi psychiatrist would have made no difference since such professionals likely had the same misconceptions about Jews as the rest of Nazi society. To truly solve the problem, the emphasis could not be on resignation; it had to be on rebellion. That is how it might have worked if even the rudiments of civilization had continued, but Hitler's madness put an end to dialogue, and to a great deal more.

Even though we live in a different country and a different time, there is much we can learn by contemplating the interaction between Nazi society and the Jews. False perceptions about minorities that begin as nothing more than distaste or a feeling of superiority can magnify to a point of separation from reality. What seemed unthinkable yesterday can become acceptable today, commonplace tomorrow and fanatical dogmatism the day after that. Both minorities and majorities can be dehumanized in the process.

Patients or Colleagues?

Be that as it may, we must deal with the problems of our own time and society (and in our case, particularly with the problems of the blind). We must do it with all of the understanding and freedom from preconception we can muster. There are still vast differences in the services offered by various agencies and volunteer groups doing work with the blind throughout the country. At the Little Rock conference to which I have already referred, this is even more apparent that it is today, and the differences of philosophy repeatedly surfaced. For instance, when blind persons come to a training center, what kind of tests do you give them, and why? In Iowa (at least this is how it was in the '60s) and in some other centers, the contention is that the blind person is a responsible individual and that the emphasis should be on his or her knowing what he or she can do. Some of the centers represented at the Little Rock conference in 1962 contended that blind trainees needed psychiatric help and counseling (regardless of the circumstances and merely by virtue of their blindness) and that the emphasis should be on the center personnel's knowing what the student could do. I asked them whether they thought services in a training center for the blind should be more like those given by a hospital or those given by a law school. In a hospital the person is a "patient." This is, by the way, a term coming to be used more and more in rehabilitation today. (That is what I said in 1962, but I am glad to say that more than thirty years later we have made a considerable amount of progress in this area.)

With respect to patients the doctors decide whether they need an operation and what medication they should have. In reality "patients" make few of their own decisions. Will the doctor "let" him or her do this or that?

In a law school, on the other hand, the "students" assume responsibility for getting to their own classes and organizing their own work. They plan their own careers, seeking advice to the extent that they feel the need for it. If students plan unwisely, they pay the price for it, but it is their lives. This does not mean that the student does not need the services of the law school. He or she probably will become friends with the professors and will discuss legal matters with them and socialize with them. From some the student will seek counsel and advice concerning personal matters. More and more the student will come to be treated as a colleague. Not so the "patient." What does he or she know about drugs and medications? Some of the centers represented at the Little Rock conference were shocked that we at the Iowa Commission for the Blind "socialized" with our students and invited them to our homes. They believed that this threatened what they took to be the "professional relationship."

Active Participation

Our society has so steeped itself in false notions concerning blindness that it is most difficult for people to understand the concept of blindness as a characteristic, as well as the type of services needed by the blind. As a matter of fact, in one way or another, the whole point of all I have been saying is just this: Blindness is neither dying or psychologically crippling. It need not cause a disintegration of personality, and the stereotype which underlies this view is no less destructive when it presents itself in the garb of modern science than it was when it appeared in the ancient raiment of superstition and witchcraft.

Throughout the world, but especially in the United States, we are today in the midst of a vast transition with respect to our attitudes about blindness and the whole concept of what handicaps are. We are reassessing and reshaping our ideas. In this process the professionals in the field cannot play a lone hand. In fact, the organized blind movement must lead the way and form the cutting edge. Additionally it is a cardinal principle of our free society that the citizen public will hold the balance of decision. In my opinion, it is fortunate that this is so, for professionals can become limited in their thinking and committed to outworn programs and ideas. The general public must be the balance staff, the ultimate weigher of values and setter of standards. In order that the public may perform this function with reason and wisdom, it is the duty of the organized blind movement to provide information and leadership and to see that the new ideas receive the broadest possible dissemination. But even more important, we must as blind individuals -- each of us -- examine ourselves to see that our own minds are free from prejudice and preconception.

Chapter 3

MANUFACTURING IDEAS ABOUT BLINDNESS

PRODUCING NEW IMAGES ABOUT BLINDNESS

In almost every society, new images about blindness are being produced. Even in economically underdeveloped countries around the world, both governmental and non-governmental organizations introduce new ideas and programs based upon these images. Several different interest groups are responsible. Among these are private agencies which create promotional material as part of their fund raising and public relations activities, and professional and interest groups who provide services to blind people. Such groups frequently update their claims for public support by providing new interpretations of the special needs of blind people. Organizations of blind people themselves provide programs and publications in which they identify incorrect and harmful stereotypes about blindness.

Of the many sources producing new images about blindness, the work of scholars and researchers receives the least scrutiny. Among those involved with blind people, scholars and researchers tend to have the highest social status and operate from a professional model that renders anyone outside their own work group unqualified to judge their results. Yet self-criticism and critiques of scientific approaches to knowledge are rare in the professional literature about blindness. In order to call attention to the harmful features in the present situation, this chapter provides detailed examples of the unreflective use of scientific methods and the selective use of materials by well-credentialed scholars publishing in reputable outlets.

SCIENCE AS THE HIGHEST FORM OF KNOWLEDGE

In most industrial societies, almost anything associated with "science" receives recognition and frequently approbation. Engineering is one arena where scientific knowledge is applied, and it has helped transform the world we live in. Each scientific success is thought to set the stage for the next "advance." The successes in the physical sciences, both basic and applied, have subsequently led social scientists to unwarranted assumptions concerning "claims of objectivity" and "truth" in their realm. For example, American sociology is dominated by scientific models of inquiry. Ted R. Vaughan (1993) has argued that this scientific sociology has unreflectively adopted a natural science model in its efforts to be scientific. The scientific method is viewed as the best and only one for producing valid and reliable knowledge because of its "objectivity." Science is considered a better way of knowing because it is based on concrete evidence and testable conclusions.

T. Vaughan argues that the scientific method and science itself is a particular form of knowledge that is historically related to the development of Western society. Rather than being objective and value neutral, science and the scientific method sometimes operate under certain assumptions about the nature of the social world that are based upon Western economic and political circumstances. Social scientists then create, observe, collect, and statistically analyze in an attempt to better understand or generalize about some limited aspect of the human condition. This so-called value neutral approach is now characteristic of all of the disciplines associated with the study of blindness and rehabilitation from special education, counseling, and testing to what is now an attempt to make the study of cane travel a scientifically-based discipline.

Philosophers have raised many questions about the objectivity of scientific information. Others have questioned the ability of humans to be value free. Although a detailed discussion of these issues is beyond the scope of this book, I will illustrate how scientific methods are violated, value positions unreflectively held, and the way "scientific" knowledge is accumulated and used to dominate discourse about blindness.

BLIND PEOPLE AS EXOTIC OBJECTS FOR ETHNOGRAPHY

An example of a recent contribution to this process is the anthro-pological monograph, *Blind People: The Private and Public Life of Sightless Israelis* (Deshen 1992). The author recognizes the distinction between the physical condition which he calls sightlessness and the more gen-erally culturally-created notion of blindness. He observes, "This usage [blindness] reflects a particular facet of Western culture: people who lack sight are not viewed by the able-bodied as merely people who have a condition of limited physical ability. Rather, they tend to be viewed as people in whose existence sightlessness is all encompassing, over reaching, total" (Deshen, p. 2). In an effort to better understand the symbolization process in which interaction is "governed" by the able-bodied, Deshen finds " . . . a rich content of attributes–beliefs, prejudices, fears–that culture has associated with sightlessness in many (perhaps most) times and places" (p.2).

Deshen thinks that blind people attract more attention than any other people with disabilities because "there is an immediate visible link between the condition and its behavioral manifestations, such as impaired mobility and lack of ability to read print" (p. 4). After describing culturally transmitted notions about blindness, he defines himself as courageous because he perceives blindness as just "an inter-esting fact of life" (p. 5). But then he says he "brought to the field a fear of blindness" (p. 9) and "prior to this project [he] had no particular interest in, or personal involvement with, blind people. But by the early 1980s, blind people struck [him] . . . as saliently exotic" (p. 8). His ethnographic study was based only on becoming acquainted with fifty-seven blind individuals in Israel (p. 7).

I question if he is really as dispassionate as he claims. He rejects the position "... of some disability-rights activists who minimize disability, trivializing sightlessness by slogans such as 'Blind people are like everybody else; they just don't see,' or 'Blindness is an inconvenience, not a handicap" (p.5). If it is more than an inconvenience, is he not endorsing the mysterious, cultural baggage idea of blindness? He reflects no awareness of the importance of the challenge that organi-zations of blind people are bringing to traditional notions about blind-ness.

Culture is not monolithic and is usually, with varying degrees of rapidity, changing. Deshen's comments about blindness leave little room for the way the definitions are being challenged and possibly changed. For example, The National Federation of the Blind has continually worked, using literature, education, litigation, and occasionally direct confrontation with agencies (reflecting "traditional" definitions of blindness), to change cultural attitudes about blindness. One possible indicator of such change is that there are now many different employment opportunities for blind people, than could have been envisioned even two decades ago. Sixty years ago in the United States, educators of blind people usually discussed employment in terms of piano tuning, making brooms and other simple tools, and sometimes even teaching other blind people (French 1932). Currently in the United States, blind people work as teachers at all levels of education and in various settings. Blind people also work as computer programmers, businessmen and businesswomen, lawyers, psychological and vocational counselors, administrators of both public and private agencies, scientists, and so forth. Blind people and others have worked to expand employment opportunities. Successful role models, campaigns to educate the general public, and the passage of laws promoting equal opportunity have led to some expansion of ideas in the United States concerning the ability of blind people to work in a wide array of occupational settings. As the remaining chapters of this book illustrate, ideas about blindness are changing under different historical and cultural influences in nations around the world. In most cases, the agencies are organizations of blind people. They are not passively dominated by culture; they are working to change some aspects of culture.

Are Deshen's biases or perhaps lack of knowledge not being revealed when he defines as "trivialities" what many people consider to be important issues? " I have little patience for some of the infighting and quibbling within the [disability rights] movement over what I feel are trivialities, such as problems of terminology, e.g., the usage of the term 'disability' in preference to 'handicap'" (p. 9). At the least, he displays a lack of awareness about the complex issues which are often very important to blind people, and he has, whether intended or not, advanced the idea that there is some quality about blindness that is more than a nuisance or inconvenience. As a scholar he has contributed the prestige of his field and his own professional accomplishments to the support of the cultural idea that there is something mysterious and dreaded inherent in blindness itself.

BLINDNESS AND CONSCIOUSNESS

In 1993, another scholar, with both an M.D. and Ph.D., published *The Strange, Familiar and Forgotten.* Israel Rosenfield uses what he calls neurological evidence to answer the question, "What is the nature and structure of our consciousness?" He writes that "traditionally, neurologists and psychologists have argued that in the classic cases, disease or trauma in the brain destroyed specific memories, or limited certain of the patient's capabilities" (p. 8). He then challenges this view: "for it is not possible to lose specific memories without profound alterations in the entire structure of an individual's knowledge" (p. 9). Regardless of the importance of the questions he raises to the field of neurology, the main source of Rosenfield's clinical evidence is a list of comments gleaned from self-reports of a few individuals who either suddenly gained or lost vision.

He offers two examples that presumably relate blindness to consciousness and perception. The first is hypothetical: if a blind man could suddenly be made to see, could he visually distinguish between a cube and a sphere? Previously, he had only experienced them by touch. The second example is a reported case of a 13-year-old boy who suddenly acquired vision when cataracts were surgically removed. The physician reports that, according to the boy, his eyes were actually "touching" the objects he now saw. They were disproportionately large and he had "no sense of distance" (Rosenfield 1993, p. 10). Subsequently, Rosenfield claims that a blind person does not develop consciousness in the same ways as do sighted people. "If a loss of visual self reference of this kind deforms a patient's sense of space, the loss of visual space itself alters the body image. This happens with blindness" (p. 64).

This author's comments about blindness, based on what he regards as clinical evidence, primarily come from the book, *Touching the Rock*, by John Hull (1990). John Hull became blind at age 24 and describes the way blindness influenced his consciousness. Dozens of blind individuals have written similar books describing their personal experience with blindness. Even when these books do not paint blindness as a tragic experience, other writers who quote them usually select "sensational" or unusual experiences. I have already described the selected use of materials in my discussion above of Tuttle's monograph, *Self*

Esteem and Adjusting to Blindness (1984). Beatrice A. Wright (1988) demonstrates what she calls the "fundamental negative bias" with examples taken from the work world of professionals in the field of rehabilitation. This bias occurs because the practitioner or researcher in the clinical or research setting is continually focused primarily on the disabling condition. According to Wright the concentration of attention results in an overemphasis upon the stigmatizing condition at the expense of many "ordinary" or otherwise positive characteristics of the individual. For me, Rosenfield is yet another such researcher who selectively uses material from a limited source to support an erroneous argument. For Rosenfield, blindness produces a restructuring of visual space and a person who becomes blind develops different images about visual space. "If a loss of visual self-reference of this kind deforms a patient's sense of space, the loss of visual space itself alters the body image" (p. 64). For his evidence Rosenfield highlights a passage in which Hull describes becoming blind at age 24.

> I feel as if I am on the borders of conscious life, not just in the literal sense that I am slipping in and out of sleep, but in a deeper and more alarming sense. I feel as if I want to stop thinking, stop experiencing. The lack of a body image makes this worse: the fact that one can't glance down and see the reassuring continuing of one's own consciousness in the outline of one's own body . . . there is not extension of awareness into space . . . I am dissolving. I am no longer concentrated in a particular location, which would be symbolized by the integrity of the body. (Rosenfield 1993, p. 64)

When Hull became blind, he lost his sense of space. "For a blind person, the loss of the visual body image initially destroys the idea of space, destroys the visual self-reference, and destroys much knowledge that is inevitably tied into them" (pp. 64-65).

I quote Rosenfield and Hull extensively lest some blind readers might think I am making this up. Unfortunately, there is more. Rosenfield continues quoting his primary "clinical" source—Hull. "Sometimes I feel that I am being buried in blindness. I am being carried deeper and deeper in. The weight presses me down. Such knowledge as I have is disappearing." The only point of reference became a body that had no extension in space: "I came back to the one thing I know. There is my body, sitting here on the edge of the bed, trembling and sweating. There is the tension in my stomach, the pounding in my temples. I hear my breathing. I feel my heart pounding. I do not know what is out there, I know what is in here." According to Rosenfield, the blind man's body image is created by internal sensations. "Hull's sense of the past is thus reduced to intimate, immediate sensations of his body in space, moving around a world he once knew in a very different way. The adventitiously blind person experiences profoundly altered subjectivity" (p. 66). Rosenfield also claims that blindness results in an altered or lost sense of time.

> But blind people are denied this perception of time as a visual relation between the individual and his surroundings; being reduced to the position of his or her own body, the blind person can judge time only by how long the body has been in motion. The blind, having no sense of the distance of physical goals, became aware of events after, not as, they happen; the world of the immediate is lost, and the world of the future is difficult to judge. (p. 66)

For Rosenfield, the brain is only understood in terms of the body in which it exists. If one loses a limb or loses the ability to process visual stimuli, the brain is also altered. "The trauma of an accident that causes blindness, for example, can (fix) visual imagery, since the brain can no longer recognize itself in the face of ongoing visual experience" (p. 135). Visual memories become disjointed and cannot be transformed by new experiences. In addition, neophysiological activities are transformed by blindness.

> The subjective sense of "deep drives and desires" are changed. For when one is blind, desires which normally bring forth images of the desired objects, feel as if dissociated from the appropriate images. Hunger and sexual desire become more abstract, less immediate. I am often bored by food, feel that I am losing interest in it or cannot be bothered by eating. At the same time, I have the normal pangs of hunger. Even whilst feeling hungry, I remain unmotivated by the approach of food. I know that it is there because somebody tells me. (p. 138)

I cannot judge Professor Rosenfield's qualifications as an expert in studying the structure of consciousness. However, I do question his judgment when he bases his arguments on a small collection of self reports by individuals experiencing physical disabilities. His great reliance on John Hull's autobiography is a clear, if unfortunate, example of how a scholar can transmit one person's experience of blindness as if he is talking about a general condition. John Hull admits to having read about twenty autobiographies of other blind people and feeling the need to write about his own "experience of blindness." I read *Touching the Rock* and can only describe it as a most unusual description of blindness. I presume Mr. Hull gave considerable thought to the symbols he chose to use. Many of them seem to come from his admitted depression or from his ideas about archetypal conditions such as light and darkness that inform his thinking. With these two men, John Hull and Israel Rosenfield, we see a compounding of the use of idiosyncratic, negative images about blindness. Hull finds a way to get his ideas published in book form. Professor Rosenfield then selects some of the most bizarre of Hull's passages to discuss blindness as a general condition and relate it to the structure of consciousness. Must it not be "truth" when a well educated scholar teaching at a reputable university in New York cites material in a book published by a major United States company? Simply put, I have had none of the experiences Hull describes. I have included a statement prepared for this volume by Gary Wunder, president of The National Federation of the Blind of Missouri and a member of the board of directors of the NFB. Mr. Wunder is a computer programmer for the medical school at the University of Missouri-Columbia. Because of his leadership experience he knows literally hundreds of blind people. I asked him to provide his response to Mr. Hull's, *Touching the Rock*:

> *Touching the Rock* stirs within me three reactions: The first is fear—fear that someone will come across this book in a library and believe it details the lives and experiences of all who are blind. The author himself is blind, articulate, and reasonably detailed. He was also once sighted and so would seem to have credibility for sighted people or the newly blind who want to learn about what life may hold without sight. The author's style of writing leaves little doubt he is stating fact. The book is full of statements which begin with phrases such as, "the blind cannot," "the blind person must," "the blind feel," "the blind are necessarily," "there is no way the blind can," etc. I have no quarrel with how the author feels, but wish he had said things like: I feel, to me blindness means, now that I am blind I can no longer, blindness forces me to, etc.
>
> The observations the author makes about the senses are made very early in his experience with blindness and many of the limitations of perception and personal interaction he experiences certainly change with time and the passage of the depression he admits. No one I know divides those with whom he is acquainted into those with faces and those without faces. No blind person I know has reported having to work at remembering that others see. None of my acquaintances have ever questioned whether they are visible because to

them others are invisible. No one I know questions his own reality because he cannot see his own face in the mirror. No one I know believes he is at the mercy of others in all of his social contacts because he is blind. Then there is the astounding assertion that blind people have less sexual desire because we can only observe one thing at a time and the sexual experience relies on a combination of stimuli to generate real excitement. As one who has been blind since birth, I am left wondering how difficult I would find my life were I to be given back all the sexual desire I have supposedly lost. What does it mean to ask whether one loses his body when he loses his visual memory? Again, this is a question I have never heard discussed among those with whom I work each day in the National Federation of the Blind.

My second impression is that this learned and articulate author did not approach blindness in the same way he would have approached any other subject about which he knew little and wanted to know much. Only one or two paragraphs were given to discussing contact with other people who are blind, and only one meeting of an organized group where feelings, problems, and solutions are discussed was ever attended. The author appears to believe the only reason for such contact would be to retreat into a world where everyone is like himself, when the reality is that organizations of the blind are not a retreat but a call to action to strengthen integration and a demand that we take concrete action to bring it about. He seems to regard adjustment to blindness as an emotional pilgrimage rather than an experience where one learns to do with other senses what he once did with vision. No one can deny the emotional adjustment blindness requires, but the space given to the difficulties and limitations of blindness remind me of the depressed patient who can think of nothing but himself and his regrettable circumstances.

My third impression is that blindness sells books, and that it is tragic so much is blamed on the lack of this sense. If a teenage child is blind and has a mental age of nine months, she will most likely be placed in a school for the blind. Does anyone who thinks ten seconds about this darling child really believe her blindness is the condition which keeps her from living normally in society? Our author writes at a time when he is admittedly very depressed. Many of his days end in exhaustion and taking to bed is a strategy he employs frequently. Even when he maintains office hours as a professor, he is still overtaken by sleep and dreams he seeks to interpret with an eye toward understanding blindness. Seeking refuge in sleep is one of the most common symptoms of depression, and yet the difficulties and limitations he describes are laid squarely at the feet of his loss of vision and the limited world to which he is now consigned. This is not to argue that the onset of blindness is seldom accompanied by depression, for quite often the two appear hand in hand, but to ascribe to blindness the mental limitations he does, leaves the reader assuming these are life-long restraints and not something which will pass as mental attitude improves.

I said earlier that I have no quarrel with the author's feelings and in fact I applaud him for being honest enough to admit them and articulate enough to express them. The fact they are expressed in a way which will reach so many makes our work to distribute another view of what it means to be blind all the more urgent.

BLIND RACCOONS

Whereas Rosenfield argued from secondary sources, images or symbols that are created, legitimated or "proved" by scientific methods are more credible in our society. According to many people, the most convincing knowledge is that reached through the empirical scientific approach. It is important to illustrate at some length how this tradition has developed within the field of blindness and to follow this with a discussion of the uncritical use of scientific methods of inquiry.

More than fifteen years ago, I read a research note entitled, "Movements of a Blind Raccoon," published in a 1969 issue of the *Journal of Mammalogy*. The article piqued my curiosity, but it always seemed a long stretch to relate a blind raccoon to current issues affecting blind people. The scientists reported that "a blind adult male raccoon (Procyon lotor) was trapped alive, radio-tagged, released 17 November 1967, and radio-tracked until killed by a trapper three months later" (Sunquist et al., 1969). Two veterinary optometrists confirmed that the raccoon had been blind due to detached lenses and glaucoma. The movements of this blind raccoon were tracked during two, one-week periods before his unfortunate demise, and were compared to the movements of a "normal adult male raccoon" (p. 145). Whenever possible, the location of each animal was determined every five minutes. Every strategy was used in an effort to follow research protocol. "Errors in estimated locations of the animals caused by unsynchronized rotation of the antennas were compensated for by a moving average of three successive fixes during periods when the animal was active and a CDC 6600 computer was used to aid in analysis of the data" (p. 145). Such scientific rigor for this one raccoon was doubtless necessary because the research, based at the University of Minnesota, was funded by the U. S. Atomic Energy Commission COO-1332-44 and the National Institute of General Medical Science.

The research findings concluded that the two raccoons, the blind one and the "normal" one, had comparable levels of activity. However, the blind raccoon traveled at a significantly faster rate than his sighted brother. "The blind animal had a lower percentage of movements at rates less than thirty feet per minute and a higher percentage of movements at rates between thirty-one and eighty feet per minute" (p. 145). The raccoons traveled through swamps and fields. The finding that surely attracted the interest of the researchers is that the blind raccoon traversed a "significantly" larger area. Not only did he travel farther, but also without apparent difficulty. "Tracks made in snow indicated that he rarely bumped into trees or other objects and these data indicate that some mechanism other than sight enabled the blind raccoon to orient within a specific area" (p. 146).

The article concludes with no further explanation of the nature of "some mechanism" which would account for the blind raccoon's ability to travel faster and farther than the control raccoon. The authors referred to the differences as significant—presumably either scientifically or statistically. This encounter with a blind raccoon and a comparison with one of his fellows was important enough to provide for yet one more contribution to scientific literature.

What about these two raccoons? Was the sighted raccoon an underachiever? Did the blind raccoon travel further and faster because of a heightened metabolic rate? I could raise sillier questions. What has anyone learned about studying two of anything when we do not know characteristics of the general population? These issues become more important when humans are involved. What does this raccoon study have to do with recent research on blindness? After a brief discussion of the notion of "best practice," I will examine issues of sample size and representativeness, the use of literature reviews, and questions of appropriateness of experimental design strategies. I argue that in the field of research on blindness, science is being narrowly defined, that important norms of science are sometimes ignored, and that a narrow focus of research interest helps create possible artificial and sometimes limiting ideas about blindness.

BEST PRACTICE

One frequently used meaning for best practice is "state of the art" or the best that we know. Since the 1940s in the field of blindness rehabilitation, we have tended to place our greatest confidence in that which is learned from "scientific studies." Occasionally, the comment is made that scientific knowledge must be linked to "common sense." However, in case of dispute or different points of view, expert knowledge based on empirical scientific inquiry is the highest or most prized information.

As any perusal of the leading journals in the field of blindness in the United States shows, empirical research follows linguistic and analytical protocol used in several academic disciplines, for example, experimental psychology. Experimental design strategies were in large part borrowed from agricultural research. Evaluation research is dominated by the largely unquestioned natural science paradigm of hypothetico-deductive methodology. This dominant paradigm assumes quantitative measurement, experimental design and multivariate, parametric analysis to be the epitome of "good" science (Patton, 1980, p. 19). To use the aura of science to legitimate claims for best practice and to apply this knowledge to programs and policy decisions about one's fellow humans conveys a great burden of responsibility.

SAMPLE SIZE AND REPRESENTATIVENESS

The July-August 1995 issue of the *Journal of Visual Impairment and Blindness* (JVIB), the leading journal in the field, illustrates several of my concerns. One issue of representativeness is raised by eighty subjects involved in a cane travel experiment (Bentzen & Barlow, 1995). Collaborators with the researchers recruited ten subjects in each of eight different cities. No explanation was given for the basis of recruitment, including the selection of cities. The representiveness of the sample is suspect because the subjects may have been recruited through existing social networks where existing practices of orientation and mobility instruction in these particular cities may have influenced the outcome. The representiveness is also suspect because 70 percent of the subjects were male. Generating ten subjects from eight different cities without a rationale adds little, if anything, to the question of sample adequacy. In the same issue, two articles are based on the study of one subject (Gerra et al., 1995).

During the period of January, 1990 through August, 1995, the *Journal of Visual Impairment and Blindness* published fourteen studies using two to four subjects and nine using only one. Should scholars attempt to generalize about the population being studied from research designs involving only one to four subjects? Surely one would not bother with the rigorous demands of scientific procedure if the results would only apply to the one or two individuals being studied.

I reviewed all of the issues of the *Journal of Visual Impairment and Blindness* since January, 1990. Table 1 presents the sample size and geographic origin of research for articles published July-August, 1995. The data presented in the chart includes only articles excluded from the table, the small number of surveys which mainly dealt with the opinions of rehabilitation professionals, family members or the general public. I also excluded literature reviews and five articles which approximated case studies.

In the four and one half years reviewed, there were nine single subject designs or quasi-design studies. Fourteen additional articles reported research on two to four subjects. As recorded in Table 1, larger sample size almost always indicated survey research design techniques and the increasing likelihood that the research was done outside the United States:

Table 1. Sample Size and Geographic Location of Research Articles in JVIB.

Sample Size	1	2 - 4	5 - 12	13 - 50	50 - Above
Number of Articles	9	14	14	39	34
Geographic Locations	US-Other	US-Other	US-Other	US-Other	US-Other
Number of Articles	8 - 1	14 - 0	11 - 3	29 - 10	25 - 9

Source: Journal of Visual Impairment and Blindness, January, 1990 through July-August, 1995

Even as sample size increased, the sampling techniques seldom yielded a representative sample. Only nine of the published studies ranging from thirty to more than nine hundred subjects involved random sampling, stratified sampling, quota sampling, or attempts to study an entire population. The remainder had sampling problems which made the results tentative at best, with no possibility of being applicable to the larger population of blind people. Perhaps the least laudable is the article, "Visually Impaired Persons' Vulnerability to Sexual and Physical Assault" (Pava, 1994). "Of the nearly 1,100 surveys that were distributed, 161 completed surveys were returned" (p. 106). The author includes a remarkable understatement: "It should be noted that this study may lack generalizability in two ways: (1) the 161 respondents may not be a random sample of the total participants at the convention, and (2) individuals who participate in national consumer conventions, such as the American Council of the Blind, may not be representative of the larger community of visually impaired persons" (p. 106).

FLAWED USE OF RESEARCH DESIGN

An article which illustrates a significantly flawed research design as well as conceptual and other questionable practices is "An Infant Sonicguide Intervention Program for a Child with a Visual Disability," by M. M. Hill et al. (1995) Despite the title's indication that the study is about a child with a visual disability, we soon learn that the subject for this study also had "significant developmental delay" (p. 329). "The subject was a five-year, four-month old boy with a congenital visual disability and significant developmental delay (he functioned at about a two-year old level)" (p. 330). There is no discussion about the relation between the "significant developmental delay" and the child's almost complete blindness. If the title of the article means anything, we conclude that the four researchers attributed the child's behavior to his near blindness and not to his developmental delay. Would a blind child without developmental disorders have performed differently?

While failing to consider this basic conceptual issue, the child's mother and the group of researchers give the appearance of following rigorous scientific protocol:

> The first two phases following baseline (Phases A & B) involved acquainting the subject with the operating characteristics of the device. During intervention Phases C through D3, a system of least prompts was used in which the trainer presented two trials using physical and verbal prompts . . . The dependent variable for the study was the number of trials in which the subject reached for and touched the stimulus objects without assistance from his mother or the experimenter. (p. 331)

Despite the authors' admitting to several additional problems, data is presented in a typical scientific format–a line graph entitled, "Percentage of Successful Trials of Assistance Level 4" (p. 334). Incidentally, the authors confess to having no adequate baseline data. Also, the mother intervened inappropriately in some cases and the research as designed was not completed. Hill et al. refer to their effort as a single subject design.

USE OF LITERATURE REVIEWS

The consequences of research based on the study of only one or two subjects are exacerbated when there is an accumulation of such studies over a period of one or two decades. The resulting long list of citations implies that a body of scientific knowledge supports the current research effort which studies one, two, or perhaps four subjects.

In their review of literature, Hill et al. (1995), in the article discussed above, cite fifteen articles related to the use of electronic travel aids. Of these, the authors mention seven studies involving intervention. The others describe different electronic devices or anecdotes from older students who have used electronic devices. Of the seven intervention studies, Strelow et al. (1978) used two subjects, Aiken and Bower (1982a) three, and their other (1982b) had eight. Later, Strelow studied four children (1983), Harris et al. reported on one child (1985), and Ferrell (1984) reviewed two earlier studies involving twenty-four children.

The article being analyzed, Hill *et al.* (1995), indicates that the results of Ferrell's two earlier studies "were not clear" (p. 330). Selective use of an article without taking into account its greater implications for the research being discussed is inappropriate. For example, Ferrell (1984) had actually presented a comprehensive review of the problems associated with young children using electronic sensory devices. It almost appears that the four authors studying this one child completely disregarded Ferrell's well-argued ethical and methodological concerns.

Most reports of environmental sensory aid use in educational programs for both early childhood and school age children have been anecdotal. Published reports are inconclusive, due either to lack of empirical data or problems in research design. Still there remains an aura around the use of environmental sensors that protects them from rigorous evaluation and criticism. Little attempt has been made to sort out individual differences in development, training or sensory utilization, and conclusions appear to be based more on personal and philosophical conviction than fact. (p. 86).

Ferrell also raises important ethical questions for researchers using human subjects:

If training is required, teachers and researchers may actually be forcing infants to discard their own methods of processing sensory information and to adopt an artificial method that is only available for part of the day and that is markedly different from the method to which they have been accustomed ... Having decided to apply intervention to an academic or social target, the researcher is confronted with these questions: Is the intervention appropriate? Is it humane? Is it the most efficient and least intrusive method to produce the desired outcome? (p. 90)

Ferrell goes on to observe that the previous nine years of research have added "little" (p. 98) to our knowledge in this area because of flaws in previous research efforts—anecdotal reports and the failure to separate out different variables which could help establish relationships among them. She then discusses five significant problems resulting from the use of binaural sensory aids. Ferrell is quite clear about one thing mentioned in both the abstract and the body of her article. "Clearly, the use of sensory aids in early childhood should be suspended until basic research into the perceptual, cognitive and motor development of blind and visually handicapped infants has been conducted" (p. 100). Hill et al. have no obligation to accept Ferrell's arguments and conclusions, but since they cite her work as a part of the tradition to which they are now contributing, they have the obligation to address the questions she raises. Had her argument been taken seriously, Hill et al. may have approached their work differently.

Despite Ferrell's cautions about research in this area, Hill and company's new study adds yet one more article using a single subject to the accumulating body of knowledge. Readers have no way of knowing if these "findings" are significantly influenced by the developmental disability. In fact, the fifteen articles cited have little if anything to do with a nearly blind child having a pronounced developmental disability. However, in the tradition of literature reviews, as we have demonstrated, uncritical readers may be impressed by an existing body of scientific research of which the current one is the most up to date.

I was one of the co-authors of the following article, which further illustrates the misuse of literature reviews. It is difficult to estimate the amount of harm done when such material as we critique is published in major journals. Incidently, the author of the article we criticize was invited to make a response. She responded but in several pages she addressed none of the questions we raise. The coauthor of the following material is JoAn Vaughan, Ph.D., Professor of Early Childhood Education at Stephens College in Columbia, Missouri.

Sex Education of Blind Children Re-Examined

This paper critiques the April, 1986, paper: "Sex Education of the Visually Impaired Child: The Role of the Parents," by Clara Shaw Schuster, published in the *Journal of Visual Impairment & Blindness*. It questions some of her assumptions of determinants of gender in early adulthood and raises questions about the imagery she uses to describe the condition of blind children. From an examination of the sources cited, we question the accuracy of her interpretation of the work of previous scholars and we suggest she has added little to the relevant literature, and through misinterpretation or misunderstanding she has presented an inadequate picture of the condition of blind children that necessitates special sex education of the type described for the parents of blind children.

Schuster's article purports to be written to help blind children in their sexual development. We fear its effect may be the opposite—that it may be detrimental to blind children, not just in their sexual development but in the social, emotional, and cognitive development as well. Schuster presents evidence based on research, but upon closer examination of her sources we find distortions and inaccurate interpretations. Consequently, the major effect of her article might be to perpetuate all too common and damaging negative stereotyping of blind persons.

In the parlance of social psychology, a stereotype is a generalization that applies to any individual who can be identified as a member of the class subsumed by that generalization. The person who holds a stereotype recognizes no requirement to test the validity of that stereotype by experience with any individual to whom it presumably applies. Implicit in a stereotype are expectations concerning the behavior of those individuals included in the generalization. One unfortunate consequence of stereotyping is that individuals often come to view themselves and have expectations for themselves similar to the stereotype, rather than what is their true potential.

Schuster's article is based upon assumptions about the limitations of blindness that are unsubstantiated by evidence. An analysis of sources cited shows inaccurate use of information given in them. Some examples from her article will illustrate why we are forced to draw this conclusion.

Schuster states that "The blind child experiences frustration at each level of development in the formation of a self-concept because the lack of vision limits both direct and indirect contact with reality." Scholl (1974), and Dickman (1975), are cited as supporting this statement. We are told that the blind child experiences frustration at each level of development. Apparently all blind children are alike, and all experience frustration at all levels of development. Any education would surely stress the uniqueness and individuality of each child—blind or sighted. Indeed, this is just what is stated in the very article that she cites. Scholl writes:

"As one reviews the potential cycle of social effects of blindness and innumerable individual and cultural variables that may contribute to how any one individual adjusts to the disability, one if forced to conclude that generalizations applied to a particular person are out of the question. Each blind person, whether child, adolescent or adults will react in his own way, out of his background of experiences and within the opportunities offered by his environment" (p. 208).

Schuster's statement contains poor educational policy when it generalizes about all blind children. However, it becomes even more damaging when it concludes " . . . the lack of vision limits both direct and indirect contact with reality." According to Schuster, all blind children can experience only a limited contact with reality. She selected a major metaphysical concept to describe interaction of blind children with their environment. They cannot know reality well because they do not experience some of its aspects visually. According to Schuster's premise, reality appears to be only that which is ultimately observed visually. By using the concept of reality with its usually profound and complex meaning, it leaves the implication of an essential deficit, not easily remedied by simple, straightforward techniques.

Later in the article, Schuster promotes another derogatory stereotype–that blindness predisposes a person to sexual maladjustment in adult life. She quotes from Foulke and Uhde (1974): "the blind child's lack of opportunity to gain experiences that inform his sighted peers, and the misconceptions resulting from this lack of experience, predispose him to sexual maladjustment in adult life." However, what Foulke and Uhde clearly point out in this same article is that the validity of this argument depends only upon anecdotal evidences:

"There has been little or none of the systematic observation that would permit an accurate description of the state of ignorance of blind children concerning sex, and no search for the relationship between such ignorance and the consequences that presumably ensue" (Foulke and Uhde).

The quote she chose was taken out of context and was the opposite from the arguments being made by the authors cited. Cooper (1984) states that:

". . . the main conclusions to emerge from studies of the blind is that although visual defect introduces considerable practical problems of daily living in areas such as travel, eating and personal care, of itself it appears not to lead to abnormal psychological development in childhood or to unsuccessful personal or social adjustment in later life."

We also question the implication that blind children have unusual misconceptions about sexual matters. Studies about children's sexual understanding show that while they often have misconceptions about sexual matters, these are not so much the result of lack of sensory or verbal information as they are the result of immature cognitive development. Unless clear evidence is found to the contrary, the misconceptions held by blind children are probably best explained and remedied in the same way as those of sighted children.

If parents and educators think that all blind children can only partially experience reality, are frustrated at every stage of development, have unusual sexual misconceptions, and are predisposed to sexual maladjustment, what are they going to communicate to blind children? How can it do other than harm their self-concept and feelings of competence? How much better for parents to assume that their blind child will develop normally and to provide sex education in ways that are natural and comfortable to the parent and child.

In this regard, we feel that Schuster places undue emphasis upon the need for providing accurate anatomical information, even if it is in ways that may be taboo to some parents. Knowledge of sexual anatomy is not as central to good sexual development as she would imply. Kohlberg's classic studies (1966) of young children's understanding of sex differences and sex roles showed that children did not use anatomical differences as the basis for determining gender. Much more important than providing anatomy lessons is the learning of positive attitudes about sexuality and having a sense of confidence and competence in interpersonal relationships. Given these, the child will find ways of learning the necessary sexual information.

Before concluding, let us make it clear that we agree with Schuster that many blind children need better sex education, as indeed do many sighted children. We disagree with her use of stereotyping and negative imagery of blind persons. She promises these while invoking the name of research evidence, though an examination of her sources shows frequent distortion and misrepresentation.

ALTERNATIVES

Several different problems have been raised in the preceding discussion. The intent is not to oppose scientific investigation or to single out a particular journal, but to suggest ways to remedy the situation described and broaden the unit of analysis on blindness-related research.

1. Researchers face a dilemma because blindness is a low incidence condition. The availability of subjects is even more limited when the incidence or prevalence of a more specific condition is the subject of research. Thus, a researcher with a curiosity about a particular condition may have only one or two cases available. The single case study has been utilized during the past hundred years on a wide array of subjects. Garmezy (1982) describes its extensive use in psychopathology, while Kazdin (1982) does question its value. "Yet the case study usually is inadequate as a basis for drawing valid inferences. Although treatment administration can be associated with therapeutic changes, the basis for these changes cannot readily be determined." However, he feels that single subject research has emerged as a valid alternative. Single subject designs have arisen, then developed into several forms of which subjects serve as their own controls, and comparisons of a subject's performance are made as different conditions are implemented over time (Kazdin, 1982). Kazdin is also quite willing to make very large assumptions about the causes of observed change: "When only the treated behaviors change, this suggests that normal fluctuations in performance and extraneous influences that are likely to affect each of the behaviors cannot account for change" (p. 42).

There is no way to control the wide array of variables which may influence the behavior or reactions of the small number of respondents. In such instances, haste makes waste, or at least the resulting information is suspect. One remedy, which would take more time but not more money, would be for the researcher to describe his or her interest in related journals or appropriate places on the Internet, and to invite researchers everywhere who might be able to involve similar subjects to participate in the project. This is widely done in well-funded medical research, in which a large number of medical schools may be involved in recruiting and studying large numbers of subjects who volunteer to try a new drug, and so forth. Even under these conditions, the samples are not randomly selected, but the resulting large number of volunteers makes it possible for their known characteristics to be compared to the known characteristics of the population in question. In the field of blindness, asking others to cooperate might not yield enough subjects to create control groups or large enough samples to permit the use of diverse statistical techniques in order to separate out the different variables possibly influencing the dependent variable. However, it would be movement in the right direction and would demonstrate to critics that we are aware of the problem.

2. The narrow focus frequently seen in published research is typical of specialization in all academic fields. However, in blindness-related research, there is frequently a narrow focus within an already narrowly limited subject area. One researcher conducts research from within the field of blindness rehabilitation, of special education, or of educational psychology, and so on, and what we end up with is a body of literature dedicated to particular attributes of blind people rather than to the broader social context of blindness. There is some evidence to suggest that being educated in the graduate programs in blindness rehabilitation and related special education programs in the United States encourages a preoccupation with traditional experimental research designs. The evidence shows this even if the number of subjects is extremely small. In fact, twenty-two of the twenty-three articles in Table 1 involving one to four subjects were conducted by researchers in the United States.

There are exceptions, but studies of blindness in other fields such as anthropology, sociology, political science and economics appear infrequently. More research from these disciplines might enable us to view blindness and blind people from a far broader perspective. Some of these disciplines more frequently use qualitative research techniques. "Qualitative data consists of detailed descriptions of situations, people, interactions and observed behavior; direct quotations from people about their experiences, attitudes, beliefs and thoughts; and excerpts or entire passages from documents, correspondence, records and case histories (Patton, 1980, p. 22). The most likely source for achieving interdisciplinary research might come from the university centers specializing in blindness rehabilitation. University teachers and researchers should encourage more collaboration among other departments and expose their graduate students to such experiences and expectations.

3. In the United States, blindness research is dominated by positivism—the search for observable facts that can be statistically analyzed to describe relationships. If an article can present "facts" which are displayed in statistical tables with sophisticated measures, it will attract more attention. As discussed earlier in this chapter, there is an ongoing lively debate among philosophers of science and scientists from many disciplines concerning the objectivity of "facts." When "facts" are proclaimed concerning aspects of individual blind people, critics may well argue that such research is not value-free and may support

existing patterns of social control. Opponents of positivism argue for a historical perspective, the use of human reason and argumentation, the need to make theoretical assumptions explicit and, in general, to raise epistemological questions about the nature of narrowly focused data analysis. Unfortunately, intellectual and theoretical debate of this type is rare in professional journals dealing with blindness. An example of this is the article by Richard Mettler, "Blindness and Managing the Environment" in *The Journal of Visual Impairment and Blindness,* 1987.

4. The problem of low incidence (there are often few cases available to be studied) could be remedied and in the long run yield more valuable information if case study techniques rather than experimental design techniques were used. Feagin et al. (1991) argue that the case study technique is indispensable to the social sciences. Orum et al. (p.2, 1991) states, "A case study is here defined as an in-depth, multifaceted investigation, using qualitative research methods, of a single social phenomenon . . . . The case study is usually seen as an instance of a broader phenomenon, as part of a larger set of parallel instances." A case study also permits the study to include the natural setting of the subject, and if some type of intervention is required, it is seen not only in a broader context but also in the ongoing history of the person or the event being studied. "An Infant Sonicguide Intervention Program for a Child with a Visual Disability" (Hill et al., 1995) would not have lacked "baseline" information if the research had been done using case study techniques. The intervention frequently associated with traditional research designs creates an artificial situation and, as Ferrell notes above, introduces unknown, possible sources of harm to the subject. Since the case study focuses on the natural setting, such an approach could avoid many of the problems encountered in Hill et al. (1995). For example, the mother mentioned in their article might have been taught the use of the particular device being studied. Researchers, by using various means, might have observed the child's behavior before the device was introduced and they could have continued to do so during and after the introduction over a longer period of time. At some point they might have been able to separate blindness from developmental disabilities in explaining the child's growth. Using a case study approach does not remove all of Ferrell's concerns about the unknown consequences of using specialized intervention devices on young children, but it would contribute more to our under-

standing than the flawed design and efforts to quantify changes in the subject's behavior mentioned above (Hill et al., 1995). Notably, during the period January, 1990, through August, 1995, only six studies in the *Journal of Visual Impairment and Blindness,* not included in Table 1, used case study techniques.

Concerning the Hill et al. study, questions of internal validity would have included a discussion of whether or not the intervention alone was responsible for behavior changes. Any number of events such as the mother's inappropriate intervention or the intrusiveness of the sonic device could have influenced the child's behavior. It is impossible to control every possible threat to internal validity. Even if the intervention has some effect on a given subject, and if we disregard previous questions of internal validity, we still know nothing from this one study concerning what might happen to other single subjects in different environments and with different physical and social histories (Tawney and Gast, 1984; Busk and Marascvilo, 1992).

SUMMARY

During the decade preceding World War II, scientific research methods were applied to the study of blind people. Subsequently, the numbers created by experimental research are seen as "objective," thus "scientific." It is assumed that numbers represent hard facts that are free from subjective values. Such studies are also regarded as "scientific" because the results can be mathematically manipulated and presented in the form of statistical tables, which carry "scientific" connotations; scientific procedures have been followed.

Research courses are usually offered in blindness rehabilitation graduate programs, and the relatively new profession invokes scientific knowledge as a primary source of legitimization. Because human subjects and clients are involved, it is imperative that the usual norms that guide scientific research be followed.

I recommend that interdisciplinary approaches be stressed to minimize a narrowly focused field committed to providing specialized services for blind people. I also suggest several different ways in which scientific research can be empirical, such as comparative research, case studies, historical research, qualitative research, and so forth, and that they be more widely used. Whenever a scientific approach is judged, it is critical that traditional norms which guide research be followed, including the use of sampling techniques, sample size, the use of literature reviews, and the concern for negative consequences for human subjects. From my review of single case studies in blindness research, my conclusion is that they demonstrate little accumulated value and do not justify the space they have been given in the primary United States journals about blindness.

As mentioned at the beginning of this chapter, the cultural images produced about blindness come from several sources. Private agencies create images, frequently intended to evoke pity, as part of their fund raising and promotional efforts. State or public agencies present information about blindness and rehabilitation to justify continuation and expansion of public economic support. Workers providing services to blind people create new explanations to justify their own occupations. Workers in academic settings, using the methods of scientific research, generate what is usually claimed to be the "most useful knowledge" about blindness.

Frequently these interest groups complement each other. Workers, through their journals and academic meetings, call themselves professionals; this enables them to claim that no one else is as well qualified as they are to make judgments about what blind people require. Professionals then lobby the government or private foundations to provide economic support to first develop and then expand specialized programs in blindness rehabilitation. Faculty, particularly those in search of tenure, must develop new ideas through published research in order to advance professionally or to keep their positions. Their departments have emerged in colleges of education or other academic units dominated by traditional models of scientific research, and the result is narrowly focused positivism.

Academic work, critical of the narrow focus of this research, is seldom published. To some reviewers of articles, papers are not even considered research if they do not contain empirical data. Cross-cultural, historical, qualitative, and other approaches to the creation of knowledge have more difficulty finding publication outlets in the United States. Speaking allegorically (Patton, 1980):

> Have you studied the experiments, the surveys and the mathematical models of the Sciences?

Beyond even the examinations, Master, we have studied in the innermost chambers where the experiments and surveys are analyzed, and where the mathematical models are developed and tested.

Still you are not satisfied? You would know more?

Yes, Master. We want to understand the world.

Then, my children, you must go out into the world. Live among the peoples of the world as they live. Learn their language. Participate in their rituals and routines. (p. 121)

BLINDNESS AND MANAGING THE ENVIRONMENT

The scientific model resulting in published research is so dominant in scholarship about blindness that theoretical articles presenting dramatically different perspectives are seldom published. The following material comes from an article by Richard Mettler, Ph.D., who works for the Nebraska Services for the Blind. This article, published in December 1987, in the Journal of Visual Impairment and Blindness illustrates a different approach to the concept of reality as experienced by blind people.

Blindness and Managing the Environment

In this paper a model is proposed for evaluating environmental modifications, advanced on behalf of blind people living in a world dominated by visual assumptions about how human beings must manage the physical environment. The first part establishes the fact that there is sound knowledge available for blind people to conceptualize and manage the physical environment on the basis of the reality of the world as known to them. The standard use in this model is the experience of a reasonable blind person trained in the skillful use of alternative (nonvisual) techniques, who possesses normal self-confidence and desire for self-direction, and who exercises care in his or her behavior. It is believed that strategies to modify the environment represent an attempt to substitute the legitimate concept-formation of the blind by concepts grounded in the visual orientation to the world in the belief that there is no autonomous and reliable nonvisual understanding of the world. In the second part of the paper, some representative examples of existing and proposed environmental modifications, the mind-set from which they emerge, and the social consequences which they will likely promote are examined in light of this model.

Subjective Experience and the Environment

In understanding how an individual learns and practices a skill, we must consider individual, subjective elements of personal skill, personal judgment and personal knowledge—*all of which are contributed by the individual in the performance.* Not only are these not formulable in formally objective terms, as is common in the language of behaviorism, they have yet to be adequately formulated through any analysis. One can describe and measure in physical terms the processes involved in human action and so detail what happens in the observable world as the behavior occurs, but of necessity this description leaves out the role of the subjective mental life of the self-directed agent. It is a fallacy to infer from the fact that you can describe human behavior in naturalistic terms, that therefore human action is adequately described.

In *Personal Knowledge* (1964), Michael Polanyi illustrates this difference by describing in naturalistic terms the behavior of a cyclist as he remains balanced on a bicycle. "When he starts falling to the right he turns the handlebars to the right, so that the course of the bicycle is deflected towards the right. This results in a centrifugal force pushing the cyclist to the left and offsets the gravitational force dragging him down to the right. This maneuver presently throws the cyclist out of balance on the left, which he counteracts by turning the handlebars to the left; and so he continues to keep himself in balance by winding along a series of appropriate curvatures. A simple analysis shows that for a given angle of unbalance the curvature of each winding is inversely proportional to the square of the speed at which the cyclist is proceeding." Polanyi then promptly rejects the formulation as inadequate because of the subjective factors left out. A physicist can tell us *what must happen in the physical world* for a cyclist to manage a turn of a given angle while traveling at a given speed, but for all its mathematical precision this does not reveal *how the cyclist manages the turn.*

This opposition between objective knowledge and subjective experience pertains to one degree or another in all skillful action. For the uninitiated, observing the performance of a skilled craftsman or artist leaves much that is unknown from that point of view. The feel of the chisel or paintbrush as it becomes an extension of the agent, subject to the agent's will, is concealed from the observer. Regardless of the activity, that which we learn through observation is different in kind from that which we learn through personal experience. Polany (1954) remarks that "Our capacity for understanding another person's actions by entering into his situation and of judging his actions from his own point of view thus appears to be but an elaboration of the technique of personal knowing . . . ." One application of this technique of personal knowing can be toward obtaining a more complete understanding of the experience of blindness.

Models of the World

Human beings have a discrete set of sense modalities through which information from the empirical world is obtained. Since the vast majority of people have access to visual information and that information predominates over information gained through other senses, the dominant model of the world is primarily vision-based. It remains the case, however, that the senses and their constitution in human beings are a biological and evolutionary contingency. It is literally an accident of nature that we acquire information as we do and so we ask: Is the sighted way of picturing the world, the sighted model of the world, the way the world really is?

There is no need for an independently established paradigm for us to realize at once that, regardless of how the world "really is," we do not have access to it. We already know that our senses set you great standards of perceptual acuity. Our auditory and olfactory capacities are but a paltry approximation of those in other animals. No one would say our capacities for taste or tactile perception are more than just enough to get by when, again, we consider how many finer examples exist in nature. Finally, we know that the human eye is sensitive to only a narrow band of radiation on the electromagnetic spectrum of frequencies. Visible light falls between the infrared and the ultraviolet. Infrared rays are too long to stimulate the retina to an impression of light, though the skin can detect their presence as heat. Ultraviolet rays are too short to perceive directly but can be recorded on photographic film.

Consider the following hypothetical case. Imagine a race of people with the same senses as we have but who can see along the entire electromagnetic spectrum of frequencies. These people would gather more empirical information from the world, have a more complete model of the world, and thereby have greater access to the way the world "really is," whatever that might mean. Two questions arise here: Could their model of the world be made accessible to us through meaningful analogs? Secondly, would we find any analogs to their model of the world useful in our management of it?

With regard to the first question, some such analogs might embody meaningful representation, however distanced from reality, by way of analog and interpretation. Imagine how we might approach an analog intended to give us some access to those features in the world which can be perceived directly only in what, for us, is nonvisible light. Perhaps we could gather some sense of what such an analog represents through a series of descriptions, analogies and a bit of mental gymnastics, but once we grasped the analog in some manner, what would we do with it? The epistemological difference is between having access to, and making use of, the *fact of nonvisible light* on the one hand and having access to *alleged phenomenological features of nonvisible light* on the other.

If we found ourselves to be a minority in a society, the majority of whom could see along the entire electromagnetic spectrum of frequencies, we would not, in their estimation, be very competent to manage the world as they found it–and they would be correct. Some of them might formulate generalizations about the seriousness of our affliction and act on an impulse to rehabilitate us. Finally, in spite of any efforts to share with us their model of the world, I suspect that some of us might stubbornly continue to manage the visual environment on the basis of our direct perception and consequent understanding of it.

Even though our senses give us no claim to an authorative access to the world as it "really is," we do manage to build from the information they provide a coherent model of the world that seems to work well enough. We are an evolutionary success, not because of the amount of specific nature of the empirical information which we gather, but because of our ability to order and make use of the information in reason and experience.

Perception Without Sight: A Personal Account

Blind people build their own model with the perceptual data at their disposal, their reason and their experience of the world. It is reasonable for them to manage the environment according to that model and not according to the common, visual orientation to the world, based on information to which they do not have access. In a contrived situation, however, sighted people can approximate the experience of the blind person's model of the world. A sighted person wearing sleepshades is at once placed in the same, immediate perceptual situation as a person who is totally blind. The following is a brief, informal account of a three-month program of sleepshade training in which I engaged.

Just as a sighted person explores the environment with the sensory apparatus available, so does a blind person, but in the latter case primarily through tactile, auditory, olfactory, and kinesthetic information gathering (supplemented by any residual vision). This initially confusing, if not overwhelming, stream of sensory data was the raw material with which I began to build a different model of the world. In time, I found that remembered visual information gradually diminished in significance as I was building this model. Most notable here was my visually dominated conceptualization of space. My working conception of space was no longer built up by considering relative positions of material objects as they appeared in my visual field. Instead, it was built up by considering relative positions of material objects separated by distances revealed through movement as I detected varying tactile, auditory and olfactory data. I then determined how objects were arranged with respect to one another, and my place among them. Familiar strategies for making visual observations, passive by comparison, gave way to strategies requiring a greater level of active interactions with the environment. The common distinction between action and observation lost much of its force as I found contacts with and manipulation of, objects in the environment more intimately connected to my observation of that environment.

Once I achieved reasonable proficiency, my use of the long, white cane as a tool became a process of probing the environment to gather information that I would normally gather visually. The auditory environment, including the various sounds produced by the cane tip as it touched different surfaces, was combined with information gathered by the shocks from the cane and the feel of the ground beneath my feet. These data were supplemented by information from noting such things as the position of the sun and wind direction and, of course, my existing understanding of the environment.

My increased awareness of nonvisual perceptual data deserves a mention. Specific combinations of different types of sensory data converged in my awareness to form a composite of data relevant to the performance of this or that task. Experience and understanding were required for me to learn first to identify, and then focus on, relevant data while I effectively ignored irrelevant data. The character of this composite which occupied my consciousness changed as I directed my attention to different tasks. Thus, the composite of data relevant to cane-traveling across a street would be built up from selected tactile, auditory and kinesthetic data. The feel of the ground beneath my feet (indicating sidewalk, grass or street); the shocks transmitted by the cane (indicating obstruction or clear path as well as the nature of the surface); the sense of the street's contours; the sounds of nearby vehicles as well as those emitted by the cane tip as it struck different surfaces; and the location of the sun or wind direction, combined to form a composite of what I needed to know in order to make a safe and efficient crossing. All of these were mutually supplementary. Awareness of, and informed selective attention to, modes of sensory data are thus central to the building of a model of the empirical world (with or without the incorporation of vision).

Some sighted people exaggerate the extent to which blind people are sensitive to nonvisual information, while others, lacking the skills to make substantial use of nonvisual data, underestimate the potential value of this information. Of course, blind people do not receive nonvisual information different from that received by sighted people. In the absence of vision, these data simply assume a coherence and usefulness with which most sighted people are not familiar. Blind people just learn to use these data more efficiently than sighted people have reason to.

In sum, I learned that just as there is a visual order and reasonableness about the world, there is an order and reasonableness which can be experienced nonvisually. One could formulate in objective terms how combinations and series of gross and fine motor movements are coordinated as tasks are pursued nonvisually. As with Polany's cyclist, however, this would only describe *what was done* and not *how the individual performed and understood what was done.* Mere observation and description, in abstraction from the experience of the self-directed agent, cannot yield a meaningful understanding of how alternative techniques are practiced skillfully in the context of the world as it is known to blind people. In the absence of this understanding, the usefulness of alternative techniques has been minimized greatly. Discussion of some specific, existing and proposed environmental modification may help to demonstrate the point.

Environmental Modifications

The understanding of blindness that leads to typical environmental modifications reflects what may be best described as the *professional's conception of blindness.* This conception has emerged from the more general *lay conception of blindness,* an amorphous collection of pre-theoretical beliefs about blindness, floating around loosely in the social mythology as articulated in the media, literature, the arts and academia. Blindness is viewed as a hardship stemming from an inability to cope with circumstances of life, including the physical environment. While the professional's conception is a refinement of the lay one, elements of both are deeply embedded in the attitudinal environment in which blind people move.

The professional's conception considers blindness generally as a technical matter reducible to a series of difficulties in negotiating the physical environment because of the absence of normal vision. Negotiating the physical world as it exists, built up as it has been according to the predominant sighted mode, *does* present certain difficulties for people who cannot see. In the application of the professional's conception of blindness, however, the nature and extent of these difficulties are exaggerated out of all proportion. The response which grows out of the professional's conception is a general effort at rendering the visual orientation to the world accessible to blind individuals through various analogues, teaching cane travel and other skills as though human action can be understood according to objectively formulated rules. The perceived technical difficulties of blindness are answered by solutions predominantly grounded in science and technology.

The conception of blindness used in this paper requires explicit recognition that blind people encounter technical difficulties in negotiating the physical environment and social difficulties in negotiating the attitudinal environment. The strategy in response to the difficulties posed by the physical environment calls for the application of human faculties to solve a problem (predominantly understanding and technique), and involves a blind person's self-directed activity as skills relevant to managing the physical environment are learned and mastered. While the built environment has been constructed with vision assumed, it *is* manageable without the use of vision.

The response to the attitudinal environment is not nearly so straightforward. Some strategies call for aggressively confronting and exposing the misconceptions about blindness found in the professional's conception. Others, as with a more thoughtful consideration of environmental modifications, can serve at least as containment measures to prevent further erosion of the attitudinal environment. The ability to move in the physical as well as the attitudinal environment has both personal and social value to blind people. The attitude that has led to typical environmental modifications places control and responsibility for movement in the world outside the blind person and within control of the greater society. This response runs counter to the most deeply held ideals of personal independence in our society.

The Architectural Barriers Act of 1968 was intended to address the problem of unfair barriers confronted by disabled people. Congress directed the federal government to set a national standard for accessibility; it soon became evident to Congress that an agency was necessary to provide assistance and enforce compliance with the law. Section 502 of the Rehabilitation Act of 1973 established the Architectural and Transportation Barriers compliance Board (ATBCB) as an independent federal agency to enforce compliance with the Architectural Barriers Act of 1968 as amended. Section 502 is applicable to most buildings and facilities constructed, renovated or maintained with federal funds.

Any study of architectural standards designed to assist blind people should include "Minimum Guidelines and Requirements for Accessible Design" (ATBCB, 1982); "Uniform Federal Accessibility Standards" (General Services Administration, Department of defense, Department of Housing and Urban Development & Postal Service, 1984) and "Providing Accessibility and Usability for Physically Handicapped People" (American National Standards Institute, Inc., 1986 [ANSI]). I will work out an ANSI in this paper. I will also draw on a number of proposed standards inspired by the spirit of the Architectural Barriers Act.

Admittedly, there is disagreement among individuals and organizations over this or that measure and its specifications. There is nothing immutable either about the standards already in place or those being proposed. Over time, existing standards will be abandoned and new ones, as well as a variety of changes in detail, will be introduced. Regardless of this flux, though, there will remain an identifiable mind-set toward blindness. The strategy inherent in each measure to be discussed is the highlighting in accessible form of an environment feature presumed to be concealed from the blind and deemed essential for competent performance. For purposes of this paper, environmental modifications will be examined in terms of the relative use-value they offer, as compared to the skillful use of existing techniques under the direct and constant control of the reasonable blind person. Also to be considered is the attitudinal impact that modifications are likely to have. While some modifications would be of some use considered in isolation from the attitudinal environment, possible benefits of a given modification must be balanced against possible detriments to the attitudinal environment in which blind people move even if the modification is judged to have some relative use-value.

It is generally agreed that blind people were realizing physical access per se long before efforts to modify the environment, but opinions are split on the degree of safety of existing access in various situations. Modifications can be usefully considered under three distinctive but frequently not distinguished categories. Some modifications are believed to introduce minimum, acceptable standards for safe access and so are tantamount to introducing physical access in practice. Some are believed simply to increase the margin of safety in existing access, and some are intended to render existing access more convenient.

While these categories do overlap, failure to maintain some clarity in a modification's use leads to confusion in its justification and adverse impact in practice.

Without clear distinctions among modifications, measures intended to increase the margin of safety or convenience tend to merge with, and gain a parasitic *prima facie* justification from, claims of disability rights to physical access per se. Such is the case with audible traffic signals. Already tested in some locations, these devices inform blind pedestrians when the standard walk-light is displayed. some audible traffic signals emit a particular bird call to inform pedestrians that east-west travel is in their favor and another bird call when north-south travel is in their favor. While this measure was intended to increase the margin of safety and convenience for blind travelers, some now propose it as a physical-access measure which introduces minimum, acceptable standards for safety and so warrants the force of law.

Audible traffic signals seem to serve a parallel function to standard walk-lights but this parallel function is less than substantive. Standard walk-lights inform motorists and sighted pedestrians simultaneously, whereas audible traffic signals inform blind pedestrians only. The most that can be said for audible traffic signals is that they might offer an additional cue for blind pedestrians to begin concentrating on commonly used strategies.

There is not much relative use-value to consider here. Pedestrian walk-lights do not signal to sighted people when it is safe to cross the street but merely when they have the right of way to cross. The pedestrian must still determine that motorists are obeying the lights direction to stop before proceeding. Audible traffic signals do not supply any information that a competently trained blind traveler cannot acquire by existing means, including the sound of vehicles idling in front, the sound of vehicles moving on either side, or the absence of all vehicle noise. Focusing on these aspects of the auditory environment informs the traveler not only that the walk path is clear but that motorists have in fact obeyed the light's direction to come to a complete stop. Not only is this a vital piece of information not obtainable from audible traffic signals, it is likely to be obscured by the sounds themselves. As it turns out, existing techniques skillfully executed by the user are the only ones that a blind traveler can use independently and safely. On the other hand, since these devices have already been deployed it is important to consider the cost they are likely to exact in the attitudinal environment.

An unmistakable suggestion is given to the community-at-large, where audible traffic signals are in place, that blind people are profoundly out of touch with their surroundings and require a mechanical aid to be aware of their surroundings. Making traffic signals audible presumes that blind people lack judgment and skill sufficient for them to negotiate street crossings with traditional signals. Almost any accommodative measure will exact some toll in the attitudinal environment, if only by reinforcing the public's tendency to interpret such devices as evidence that blind people as a class do not possess the abilities commonplace among sighted people. Prospective employers—doubtful that a blind applicant can consistently arrive at work on time, let alone satisfy all job duties competitively—will not abandon those doubts when presented with the seeming necessity for an elaborate accommodation, simply so a blind person can cross a street safely. since there is no relative use-value when considering the probable impact on the attitudinal environment, this measure will yield for blind people a net loss in social utility. Movement in the physical environment will not be enhanced, and movement in the attitudinal environment will become more difficult.

Many modifications are proposed in the name of bringing access to mass transit facilities up to a reasonable standard of safety, as in the following examples: safety barriers between subway cars to prevent blind people from stepping between and falling through two cars, as with the R-44 and R-46 subway cars used by the New York Metropolitan Transit Authority; audible indications above mass-transit car doors to inform blind people of the location of available entrances; and textured or otherwise tactile warning strips affixed to the ground to warn blind people of their proximity to the edge of a subway platform. These proposed measures, however, offer nothing that is not already available through competent cane technique. Spaces between cars, entrance ways, and changes in level are precisely the kinds of environmental features that cane technique is intended to detect. The traveler, having detected these features, interprets the information and directs his movements accordingly. Further, it seems unlikely that audible door indicators would provide more auditory information than is typically provided by doors opening and closing and other available sounds. In the case of particularly quiet subway trains, some marginal use-value might occur in reducing slightly the time taken to find an available entrance. On the other hand, movement in the physical environment would not be enhanced to a significant degree, and movement in the attitudinal environment will become more difficult, given the likelihood of the public's generalizing from this statement on the blind population's alleged incompetence to other areas of imagined incompetence.

The following standards from ANSI also purport to bring margins of safety up to an acceptable level:

4.7.7 Warning Textures. "A curb ramp shall have a detectable warning texture . . . extending the full width and depth of the curb ramp, including any flares."

4.7.12. Uncurbed Intersections. "If there is no curb at the intersection of a walk and an adjoining street, parking lot or busy driveway, then the walk shall have a detectable warning texture . . . at the edge of the vehicular way."

4.27.5. Detectable Warnings at Hazardous Vehicular Areas. "If a walk crosses or adjoins a frequently used vehicular way, and if there are no curbs, railings or other elements . . . separating the pedestrian and vehicular areas, the boundary between the areas shall be defined by a continuous "thirty-six-inch-wide tactile warning texture."

4.27.4. Detectable Warnings at Stairs. "All stairs, except those in dwelling units, in enclosed stair towers, or set to the side of the path of travel shall have a detectable warning at the top of stair runs."

4.27.3. Tactile Warnings on Doors to Hazardous Areas. "Doors that lead to areas that might prove dangerous to a blind person (for example, doors to loading platforms, boiler rooms, stages and the like) shall be made identifiable to the touch by a textured surface on the door handle, knob, pull or other opening hardware."

4.27.6. Detectable Warnings at Reflecting Pools. "The edges of reflecting pools shall be protected by railings, walls, curbs or detectable warnings."

Tactile warnings are not likely to advise a traveler of anything but their own presence. The great variety of environmental situations which call for their application also call for a variety of responses. A traveler relying on tactile warnings to any considerable extent has to reflect upon what any particular one is intended to indicate and thereby divert his or her attention from more informative and valuable nonvisual information. Tactile warnings would not be reliable, because only a small fraction of the environment is subject to these standards. Even when subject to them, it would be unwise for a traveler to infer anything from the absence of a tactile warning in any given situation. Dependence on tactile warnings thus entails relinquishing control and responsibility for self-directed action according to one's own experience in favor of the judgement of others. For the reasonable blind person, tactile warnings will amount to peripheral environmental data which lack any real, functional relevance and must continually be filtered out of the composite of data which can be acted on with confidence.

An extreme case of this can be found with what are known as "Pathfinder Tiles." These tiles—made of various tactile materials, such as synthetic rubber, vinyl, concrete or ceramic clay—are considered by some to be the best way of providing surface tactile information. They come in two forms, one-half-inch-high dots, intended to serve as warnings at the kinds of locations cited in ANSI, and one-half-inch-high bars, to guide travelers in a straight line such as when making street crossings. It has also been suggested that the bar form be used to guide blind people through public facilities.

The bar form constitutes a significant move beyond even tactile warnings. A traveler relying on the bar form is encouraged to travel from point to point assuming that this path will not lead to any danger or inconvenience. Again, however, the traveler encountering bar tiles must still determine what path they form. As with warning tiles, encountering bar tiles still requires the traveler to engage in further information-gathering to decipher what the tiles signify. This further information-gathering provides the data necessary to make rational decisions about how to direct one's actions, bypassing altogether consideration of the tiles. Since blind people are capable of determining on their own what these tiles signify (and must do so to insure their safety), merely encountering them serves no clear purpose.

The following standards, proposed as safety measures, are more reasonably understood as matters of convenience:

4.4.1. (Protruding Objects) General. "Objects protruding from walls (for example, telephones) with their leading edges between 27 in. and 80 in. above the finished floor shall protrude no more than 4 in. into walks, halls, corridors, passageways or aisles." . . . "Free-standing objects mounted on posts or pylons may overhang 12 in. maximum from 27 in. to 80 in. above the ground or finished floor. Protruding objects shall not reduce the clear width required for an accessible route or maneuvering space."

4.4.2. Headroom. "Walks, halls, corridors, passageways, aisles or other circulation spaces shall have 80 in. minimum clear headroom. If vertical clearance of an area adjoining an accessible route is reduced to less than 80 in. . . . a guardrail or other barrier having its leading edge at or below 27 in. above the finished floor shall be provided."

In many circumstances, the sound of the cane tip striking a hard surface will echo and so advise the traveler of an overhang. Where the floor is carpeted or for whatever other reason no echo can be heard, low-hanging obstacles are a nuisance and this kind of modification would eliminate the occasional bump on the head at facilities subject to this standard. This would probably be appreciated by everyone but the motivation is to care for blind people. The reason 27 inches is the stated maximum allowable height above the floor in the previous standard is that, even when exercising competent cane technique, a traveler is not likely to contact an object resting above that distance from the floor. This might generally be true, but bumping into objects from time to time is just one of the innumerable inconveniences with which we are all confronted. For society to apply the force of law to reduce the incidence of this minor inconvenience for blind people is tantamount to declaring them too fragile to negotiate the most insignificant of life's irritations.

The final category of modifications and measures includes those proposed simply to increase convenience for the blind, such as the placement of furniture and other items in order not to obstruct likely paths of travel. These measures can be dismissed for the reasons already discussed. Other measures concern various forms of access to the kinds of information made available to sighted people. Many such measures would be acceptable on grounds of attitudinal impact. ANSI contains modifications such as tactile control indicators on elevators, increased illumination levels around and in elevators, raised or indented characters and symbols on elevator panels, and color contrasts between characters and symbols and their backgrounds. Proposed measures from other sources include specifications for other types of signs, graphics and information display—such as tactile and auditory maps, talking elevators, talking signs and prerecorded instructions for a variety of other information purposes.

Elevators can present difficulties, since there is a variety of panel arrangements. Once familiar with a particular elevator, blind people have no further need for assistance. Since they can be expected to encounter all manner of panels, however, the simplest solution for most people might be talking elevators. Common, laminated signs with raised or indented letters have been found useful, as have tactile characters and symbols and Braille displays. Talking signs and other prerecorded information might also have a place in particular situations. As it turns out, the measures which keep focus of control within the blind person and assume judgment and skill tend to be simple and discreet, and are often attitudinally neutral or nearly so. Of course, when all else fails, blind people do what the rest of us do when we require information—they ask someone.

Neoinstitutionalization

Environmental modifications on behalf of blind people represent a new form of institutionalization, a tangible extension of a vestigial institutional mentality toward blindness in the greater society. This new form may properly be called "neoinstitutionalization."

The mind-set from which one provides physical, social or political access to another is one of fairness and social justice. The mind-set from which one assumes responsibility for the safety and convenience of another is custodial, and of necessity must be supported by beliefs about a basic lack of ability in that other person. Two mind-sets merge and complement one another in an institution as a social order is established and maintained, namely, a custodial mind-set and a compliant and dependent mind-set. The residents in a benevolent institution are surrounded by a safe and convenient environment in which little is expected from them and a great deal is done for them. The resident's decisions are few and limited; the institution's decisions on his or her behalf are many and significant. At every turn, control is outside the resident.

The forces at work in instilling compliant modes of behavior are formidable. Residents are encouraged to think of themselves as incompetent and rewarded for behaving accordingly. The resident who internalizes this understanding imposed by others must at once deny his or her potential as fully capable, fully participating, independent adults and place his or her destiny as a human being in a judgement of those others.

The effects of the current attitudinal environment are felt by blind people in various ways. Many blind people are denied jobs or promotions out of hand with no serious consideration being given as to how they might do the work. Blind young people are often denied educational opportunities out of the conviction that they cannot do the same work as sighted students. There can also be subtler, yet no less dehumanizing forms, such as when one rushes to open a door, offers unrequested directions or indeed, imposes any of the hundreds of other kinds of unsolicited assistance out of the conviction that a blind person could not manage without this assistance. All of this individually and collectively chips away at the recipient's sense of humanity.

No one pretends that environmental modifications can realistically be put into place on any comprehensive scale, yet their proponents maintain that at least some modifications are necessary for blind people to have access to facilities competently and safely. The result for blind people who have not had the kind of training which promotes the attributes ascribed to the reasonable blind person will be an archipelago of secure and convenient islands–mini-institutions–within the greater society. From home to the local federal building and back, the blind person may feel at ease, for his convenience has been arranged by others, but this sense of security is hollow in an artificial environment. For a blind person who has internalized the need for such accommodations, full, independent access to the unmodified environment must ever remain something to which he or she dare not aspire.

The irony of this is that the strategy of environmental modifications designed to contribute to the social integration of blind people will in fact act as a barrier to their social integration. Environmental modifications, advanced in the name of increasing the independence and integration of blind people, threaten to contribute to their dependence and isolation by reinforcing the belief that blind people are, by nature, inherently incompetent. The inescapable social consequence of this general belief is a reduction in opportunities for participation and success in most important areas of human endeavor.

Chapter 4

BLINDNESS IN THE UNITED STATES: FROM ISOLATION TO FULL INCLUSION

C. EDWIN VAUGHAN AND JOAN VAUGHAN

Blindness in the United States can only be understood in terms of the influential European cultural traditions combined with more recently developed programs and policies. The cultural traditions have their origins in ideas and arrangements borrowed from England, France, Austria and other European countries. In turn, these have their roots in religious values and social arrangements which appeared first in early Judaism and later in Christianity and Islam.

CULTURAL ORIGINS OF BLINDNESS IN ANTIQUITY

Blindness is frequently described in early Greek drama. It was sometimes inflicted on individuals or on entire groups, such as residents of a besieged city or members of a captured military unit as punishment. In this chapter, I draw heavily on the work of Berthold Lowenfeld, particularly his monograph, *The Changing Status of the Blind* (1975). His survey of the cultural roots of blindness in the West is more comprehensive than most, and it benefits from sources not available to me. Either they have not been translated into English or they are rare.

In ancient Greece some blind individuals were notable as poets, teachers, or fortune tellers. However, many were beggars, while others were segregated to perform repetitive tasks, including working in mines. Reported for the first time in ancient Greece were special sup-

89

port programs for blind people. Solon of Athens wanted to help blinded war veterans, and a tradition was begun which persists to this day.
"At first, the law furnished assistance only to those who had become
blind or crippled as a result of war, but later it was extended to civilian invalids also. The amount of money that they received is said to
have covered about half the cost of modest living" (Lowenfeld, 1975,
p. 21). One had to be a citizen of Athens and own some property in
order to receive these benefits. Almost exclusively, blind beggars
came from families who were already poor. In general, the elite in
Greek and Roman societies had no public concern for social justice.
"Plato stressed the love of beauty in his dialogues, and in his Republic
the warrior ranked next to the philosopher in importance and prestige.
These ideals implied a rejection of their opposites—infirmity, inability
to fight and deformity" (p. 24). The rare programs, such as Solon's policy in Athens, were not typical of early Greek and Roman societies.
Those who could not sustain themselves had no claim on society.

Compassion for the less fortunate was the contribution of Judaism,
Christianity, and Islam. "The spirit of 'aren't we all children of one
God' is inherent in monotheistic religions, but it took some time to
change distrust of strangers and the strange, to the point where they
were accepted into one's house and treated like family" (p. 25).
Israelites were enjoined not to put a stumbling block before the blind,
nor to lead them astray (Leviticus 19:14 and Deuteronomy 27:18).
"The comments on blindness in the Bible are generally made within
the context of commiseration and compassion and not with the con-
tempt or revulsion that we often find in Greco-Roman literature"
(p. 27).

In Europe, economic and social conditions were in decline even
before the fall of the Roman Empire in 476 A.D. The first organized
efforts by the Christian church led to the establishment of hospitals.
The first hospital (Xeuodochium) was founded in 369 in Asia Minor.
"It resembled a town in which special sections were set aside for every
kind of people in need and it was well organized. Blind people were
also admitted" (p. 35). Later, hospitals exclusively for the blind were
also established. In 1254, King Louis IX built one of the best known
hospitals, which served three hundred men blinded during one of the
Crusades. Such hospitals did not escape criticism, as Lowenfeld notes
in citing a German source: "I do not know why the king has assembled 300 blind people in one house. They roam in bands the streets of

Paris and do not cease to shout while the day lasts. They push each other and inflict on each other contusions because nobody is there to guide them" (p. 36).

Hospitals and religiously-motivated charities met the needs of only a small portion of blind people. Beggars of all types, including the blind, were seen as a public nuisance. However, a different type of public response, not based on religious sentiments or charity, developed in England late in the sixteenth century. Following the defeat of the Spanish Armada in 1588, the English government established a hospital to provide care for members of the Royal Navy in case of injury, sickness, or old age. This hospital was maintained by funds withheld from the monthly wages of the seamen. Thus, during an era when extremely punitive measures were being directed toward the disabled and the poor, England established a program of compulsory health and disability insurance for a category of citizens on whom the welfare of a society at large was thought to depend (Strauss, 1966, p. 6).

When aid from the church was inadequate or not forthcoming, blind people began to create their own organizations. Brotherhoods or guilds were formed to protect the interests of their members. By the sixteenth century they existed in France, Germany, England, Russia, and several Asian countries (Vaughan & Vaughan, 1994, p. 41). Guilds developed for almost every craft, and membership was usually obtained through apprenticeship. Although economic issues were paramount, guilds also addressed social and philanthropic concerns. Guilds flourished because governments were unable or unwilling to protect the interests of citizens. Those of blind people, like those of beggars, reflected the organizational patterns of other guilds. They were self governing, based on group interest and involved apprenticeship (see Chapter 5 for a more detailed description of guilds in China and Chapter 7 for those in Spain). Guilds determined where and how their blind members would beg.

Of course, guilds and religiously-based charities did not prevent large scale poverty; governments also began to respond. France passed a poor relief tax in 1554. Similar developments culminated in the Elizabethan Poor Laws of 1601. "Justices of the Peace had to appoint two to four overseers of the poor who were chosen from the most respected citizens of the community" (Lowenfeld, 1975, p. 43). By the seventeenth century, the West now had three major traditions which persist to the present: religiously-based concern, secular-based concern and the tradition of "noblesse oblige," the inferred obligation of people of high rank or social position to behave nobly or kindly to the less fortunate.

During the sixteenth century, a small number of blind people became educated and demonstrated their ability to the wider society. As early as 1526, Vives described activities of blind people in Spain:

> Nor will I suffer the blind to sit around or wander about idly; there are a large number of things in which they may be active; some are suited to the sciences, let them study, in some of these we see a progress of erudition not to be belittled; others [are suited] for the art of music, let them sing, let them play upon the strings, let them breathe into the flutes; let others turn the lathe or the little wheel; let others draw the wine press. (cited in Lowenfeld, 1975, p. 45).

In the seventeenth and eighteenth centuries, several blind people distinguished themselves by obtaining advanced levels of education. Lowenfeld gives brief biographical sketches of more than thirty blind people for their cultural attainments, despite blindness (1975, pp. 49-63). He observes that so many self-emancipated blind people appeared partly because of the general increase of literacy in Europe. Prominent French writers including Diderot, Voltaire, and Rousseux helped create curiosity about the potential of blind people. In his most influential writing on education, Emile Rousseux urged the sighted to imitate the blind: he wanted them to possess the advantages that the blind possessed in darkness. "[W]hy, then are we not given practice at walking as the blind do in darkness, to know the bodies we may happen to come upon, to judge the objects which surround us–in a word, to do at night without light all that they do by day without eyes?" (1762, p. 133). Subsequently, enlightenment ideas concerning human reason, freedom and humanitarianism enriched the cultural environment experienced by blind people.

Valentin Haüy established the first school for the blind in 1784, and King Louis XVI was so impressed by this school that he contributed funds for it.

> Twenty pupils, all of them blind since birth or infancy, read out loud from books specially printed in raised relief-print, identified places and features on maps, sang and played musical instruments in his honor. The older children were also able to set type, spin yarn and knit hose. Especially impressive was

an eleven-year-old boy, Le Sueur, who had been the first of Haüy's pupils, discovered pathetically begging for himself and his seven brothers and sisters and
who now was the prodigy of the class, almost a teacher in his own
right. (Schama, 1989, pp. 188-189)

In the preparations he made for starting the first school for blind
children, Haüy realized the necessity of a suitable means for reading
and writing—an approach based on touch. He involved his students in
experiments with embossed, raised print. However, progress in this
area awaited the insight of a blind French citizen, Louis Braille (1809-
1852), who recognized the advantages of raised dots over palpable line
lettering. Haüy's school also started the tradition which persists to this
day: that schools for the blind should both educate and prepare students for work.

From 1791-1799, four schools were founded in England, two of them
by blind men. Johann Wilhelm Klein founded the first school in
Austria in 1804. This school proved important as a model for others
because Klein believed that the blind should be the responsibility of
the government, not charity. "This led Klein to the conclusion that the
solution for the problems of providing education for every blind child
was in their placement in local public schools" (Lowenfeld, p. 81).

SCHOOLS FOR THE BLIND IN THE UNITED STATES

The first schools for blind children in the United States opened their
doors in 1832. These were the Perkins School for the Blind (first incorporated in 1829 as the New England Asylum for the Blind) and The
New York Institute for the Education of the Blind. Through the leadership of Samuel Gridley Howe, the Perkins School quickly emerged
as a national leader for the education of blind children. The origin of
Perkins and many of its subsequent developments were directly influenced by schools for the blind in Europe. In 1824, a Boston physician,
Dr. John Dix Fisher, visited L'Institut National Pour les Sueugles (The
National Institute for Blind Youth) in Paris (Stuckey, 1996). There he
saw blind students studying ancient and modern languages, music,
reading and writing, manual vocations, mathematics, and geography.
"On his return to Boston in 1826 Fisher reported on how similar institutions, or as a number of them were called at that time, *asylums,* for

the blind had been established in other European cities such as St. Petersburg, Vienna, London, Liverpool, Edinburgh, Dublin, Bristol and Norwich" (p. 9). The word "asylum" at this time had a positive connotation: students were being rescued from the bedlam of work-houses, almshouses and mental institutions and provided their own special place. Having resolved to develop a school for blind children in the United States, Fisher approached several wealthy Bostonians for financial support. His efforts culminated with the opening of what became the Perkins School in 1832.

Fisher had been acquainted with his fellow physician, Samuel Gridley Howe, before each of them had parted to spend several years in Europe. In 1831, Fisher and the Perkins trustees offered Howe the opportunity to become director of the proposed new school. Howe immediately spent a year visiting schools for the blind in different areas of Europe. He was critical of the approach used by some of the state-sponsored schools and also noted that "other institutions sup-ported by individuals and public benevolence tended to overprotect their pupils and to treat them as objects of charity" (Stuckey, 1996, p. 10). However, Howe did hope to incorporate their best features:

1. Each child should be considered as an individual and should be trained according to his or her abilities.

2. The curriculum should be similar to that of the public schools. It should be well-rounded, but might include more music and crafts than did the public schools.

3. Blind students should be trained to become full participants in and con-tributing members of their home communities. (Farrell, 1956, p. 88-89)

The first two teachers employed by Howe came to Boston from the schools in Paris and Edinburgh (Lowenfeld, p. 89).

Howe neither met nor apparently knew about Louis Braille. Instead, the three leading United States schools, one each in Boston (Perkins), New York City (Lighthouse), and Philadelphia (Overbrook), compet-ed for more than four decades to develop embossed reading systems. Howe absolutely rejected the Braille System being developed in Europe. As a result, a polarized struggle was carried on between blind teachers and sighted administrators and teachers in the United States.

Blind teachers consistently favored the dot system over embossed lines. This conflict over Braille also developed in Europe (Farrell, 1956, p. 100). Although the School for the Blind in Paris adopted what came to be known as the Braille System in 1854 (Lowenfeld, 1973), it was not until 1916 that it was widely accepted in the United States.

Howe was consistently ahead of others in his concern about the possible harmful consequences of segregating blind children. He thought that schools were needlessly regimental and pushed blind students into a common mold. He saw the importance of cottage or small group housing, and he was among the first in the United States to argue that blind students, whenever possible, should remain in the home and neighborhood schools. Howe stated in an 1866 speech, "I am constantly applied to by teachers as to how to proceed with a blind child; and I always encourage them to keep it at home and let it go to the common school as long as possible" (Stuckey, 1996, p. 12).

SHELTERED WORKSHOPS

In the nineteenth century, educators of blind people failed to anticipate societal resistance to the employment of their students. Graduates of schools for the blind could not find jobs. "Thus, educators of blind people became disillusioned and abandoned goals of equality and integration because they could not place their graduates in competitive employment" (Vaughan, 1993, p. 174). Early educators had hoped that blind children, as a part of their education, could be taught occupational skills that would enable them to maintain themselves.

> Sheltered workshops, as such, first arose in America over a century ago as an outgrowth of the special schools for the blind whose curricula concentrated upon the provision of simple forms of vocational training -- in such limited and manual skills as weaving, knitting and chair caning, as well as in music and similar arts. (tenBroek, 1962, p. 21)

Jacobus tenBroek observed that several different historical traditions influenced present-day sheltered workshops in the United States. Religious organizations had, for centuries, provided protection and other services for some blind people. These organizations usually had the spiritual well-being of blind people as their main concern. Sheltered workshops run by the Salvation Army, according to tenBroek, exemplify this tradition. Second, and often related to religious organizations, medieval hospitals fed and cared for the sick, nourished and raised abandoned infants and orphans, confined the insane, and housed the blind.

> Those present-day workshops which incorporate the provision of medical and therapeutic services therefore may be seen as the outcome of a line of development reaching back to the medieval hospital and extending through the American country hospitals of more recent times—institutions which also sought to fulfill the "double   function" of healing the sick and employing the handicapped. (tenBroek, 1962, p. 23)

The almshouse, or workhouse, developed as a secular arrangement to provide a different kind of service. The chief importance of the workshop was not care of the sick or disabled, but to provide employment to the able-bodied poor. Conditions were often harsh and wages low. Another tradition was the nineteenth century workshop developed as an adjunct to the schools to educate blind children. "However, it is significant that these schools soon deliberately severed their connection with the shops they had themselves created, as it became apparent that the functions of education and employment could not feasibly be mixed within the same program" (pp. 22-23).

Eventually, workshops came to be operated independently from either custodial or educational institutions. Workers in these shops, with very few exceptions, were not eligible for unemployment compensation, nor did they, until recently, have the right to collective bargaining. The justification was that the purpose of workshops was rehabilitation and any commercial activity was a part of the rehabilitation process. In 1962 tenBroek observed:

> [T]he greatest deprivation to workers in sheltered workshops is the exemption of those shops from the minimum wage provisions of the Fair Labor Standards act. With reference to the blind alone, at least 85 of the more than 100 sheltered shops primarily employing sightless workers hold certificates of exemption issued by the Department of Labor under Section 214 of the act. (p. 29)

In 1960, the average wage paid in sheltered workshops was .53 cents per hour while the national minimum wage was $1.00 per hour. Today many sheltered workshops pay at least the minimum wage.

Scott (1967) studied changes that occurred in the management of sheltered workshops and illustrated how organizational interests created conditions frequently seen as contrary to the interests of blind workers. As workshops became larger, management and marketing concerns became dominant. Ordinary business concerns frequently prevailed over rehabilitation concerns. Scott used the concept of goal-displacement to explain how daily policy decisions of organizations could modify and sometimes subvert their original goals. He also analyzed material from the annual meetings of the American Association of Workers for the Blind. For example, a survey of workshops conducted in 1935 reported that it was undesirable to employ workers older than 45. "When we take into consideration the months and even years that it takes to train a blind person to be a top notch producer, we realize that any higher age limit would tend to reduce the years of usefulness to such an extent that it might well be a losing proposition" (AAWB Proceedings, 1935, p. 83). Most workshops ignored employee complaints. Some managers and their boards of directors were simply unwilling to concede any power or economic improvement to blind workers. "Regardless of institutional affiliation, the director of a rehabilitation program is accountable to multiple public, private and corporate constituencies as never before" (Albrecht, 1992, p. 189).

Most early workshops trained their students to produce craft items, particularly brooms of all types of sizes. This ensured that workers in the early shops were not competing in the general labor market. A new institution had been created: a place where blind people could work and a place where the type of work was suitable for blind people.

There were occasions when workshops developed independently of schools and previously existing institutions. For example, early in the twentieth century a group of citizens from Memphis, Tennessee, became interested in the plight of blind people and began to lobby for a publicly funded program. In 1917, these efforts led to the legislation that created the Tennessee Commission for the Blind, and in 1918, it established a workshop separate from the School for the Blind. Initially, much of the work, particularly that of women, was done in each person's home. Unfortunately, at the end of the first year of the Commission's work, it was reported that 40 women were doing poor quality piece work in their own homes. "As a result of their eagerness to work, their reluctance to give it up when once started, and their inability to do anything but very plain sewing, we have stocked up almost too heavily on aprons and towels" as (cited in Coleman (1947, p. 4). During this same first year, 10 blind men earned a total of $1,095.14 for their labors at broom making, or 60 percent of the $1,737.38 income generated by their ability.

In 1918, graduates from the Tennessee School for the Blind were demanding that at least one blind person be on the Board of Commission for the Blind. As a result, D. M. Coleman was appointed in 1919 to be the first blind member of the Tennessee Commission; subsequently, he became its Executive Secretary. His report for the period 1920-1922 indicated that the number of workers had more than doubled, from 19 to 45.

> Many of the men coming to our shop have lost their sight as a result of pre-mature explosions or other accidents, after they had passed thirty years of age. They came to us with active bodies and having been accustomed to the use of tools and being now taught to substitute the sense of touch for that of sight, they soon became skilled mechanics, supporting their families and in many instances earning more than they received before the accident which deprived them of their sight. (Coleman, p. 12)

In 1923, Mr. Coleman was elected to the Tennessee legislature, but he continued his lifelong interest in the Tennessee workshop. Apparently, it was a source of pride for Mr. Coleman and his successors that many of their workers earned as much as comparable sighted workers or as much as they had earned before they became blind (p. 23). Eventually, the Tennessee workshop employed a blind person to be in charge of sales, which demonstrated to many that a blind person could be as good a salesman as anyone else. In the annual report, Mr. F. R. Morton noted that the Tennessee workshop had become the largest in the United States for making brooms, and that it employed both men and women.

There are now more than one hundred sheltered workshops that provide employment primarily for blind people, including workers with multiple disabilities and vision loss. Some of the contradictions within these organizations are analyzed in Hope Deferred by Jacobus tenBroek and Floyd Matson (1959). Could an organization that frequently had to be seen as an economically rational business also have as a goal the rehabilitation of workers and their placement in competitive employment? Were these workers being exploited? Were they receiving a fair share of the revenues generated by their labor? In 1918, as mentioned above, the Tennessee workshop appeared proud that sixty percent of the revenue generated was paid to workers. However, as the decades unfolded, workshops became more organizationally complex and diversified in their products. The National Industries for the Blind (NIB), discussed below, became the means of channeling government contracts to affiliated workshops across the United States. A percentage of all workshop sales went to the NIB for new product development, adaptive equipment development, and the overhead of the national organization. As reflected in the annual reports of the NIB, the percentage of revenue going to workers' salaries declined from decade to decade.

Additional recurring questions have since arisen: Do blind people have opportunities for upward mobility within workshops? Is the pay of workers low relative to the salaries of administrators, who are usually not blind? Should workshops be allowed to pay workers less than the minimum wage because they are not regular workers but people receiving "rehabilitative services"? Should blind workers be allowed to organize labor unions to pursue their common interests? Are workshops useful at all when they are "dead-end" areas of noncompetitive employment? All of these questions have been concerns reflected in the consumer literature of the National Federation of the Blind.

AGENCIES AND PROFESSIONS

If schools for the blind attracted the most attention in the nineteenth century, the first decade of the twentieth century witnessed the rapid emergence of private agencies. At the turn of the century there was almost no employment for blind people outside sheltered workshops. The labor force in urban areas continually received new waves of immigrants eager to work. As a result, the following multipurpose agencies developed in major United States cities: the New York Association for the Blind (1905), the Chicago Lighthouse for the Blind (1906), the Cleveland Society for the Blind (1906), the Buffalo (New York) Association for the Blind (1907), the Albany Association of the Blind (1908), the Maryland Workshop for the Blind (1908), the Cincinnati Association for the Blind (1910), and the Massachusetts

Association for Promoting the Interests of the Adult Blind. Such privately supported programs were frequently established with the special purpose of attracting the interest of local philanthropists. For example, two sisters, Winifred and Edith Holt, founded the New York Association for the Blind in order to distribute theater tickets to blind people. The Cleveland Society, formed in 1906, included programs for the prevention of blindness, treatment for eye disease, literacy, placement of blind children in public schools, and the production of brooms, rugs, and baskets in a sheltered workshop. It also offered information and referral services.

> Nearly all of these agencies also provide direct aid to the poor and infirm blind incapable of learning a trade, friendly visiting services to alleviate the loneliness of the blind (later home teacher services), sales opportunities for homemade products, entertainment and recreational facilities, and public information services "to arouse the public to a clearer appreciation of the capabilities of the blind." (Lowenfeld, 1975, p. 277)

In almost all cases, these agencies were governed by a board of directors whose members were usually either wealthy or influential. Fund raising was often based on public appeals, openly evoking pity for the recipients of charitable contributions. For example, in a speech entitled "In Aid of the Blind" delivered to the New York Association for the Blind at the Waldorf-Astoria, March 29, 1906, Samuel Clemens (Mark Twain) said, "Now it is dismal enough to be blind; it is a dreary, dreary life at best, but it can be largely alleviated by finding something for these poor blind people to do with their hands" (Clemens, 1910, p. 324). Unfortunately, ninety years later, I have often observed fund raising appeals using the same extremely negative images of people who happen to be blind or somehow disabled. As one might guess, blind people were infrequently employed in these agencies.

The next major growth in services for blind people came from the federal and state governments in the United States. Sympathy for blinded war veterans following World War I led to funding and cooperation between federal and state agencies. In 1920, President Wilson signed the Smith-Fess Act, which led to a $750,000 appropriation in 1921 for a joint federal-state program of vocational rehabilitation for the physically handicapped. Thus began the flow of federal money which has become a major economic resource for the blindness rehabilitation system. In part, the Act reflected a broad base of concern for blinded World War I veterans, and the establishment of the Federal Board of Vocational-Education has gradually led to the jointly funded federal-state rehabilitation program of today.

> When the first war blinded soldiers of World War I returned to the United States, they were admitted to Evergreen, a United States Army General Hospital in Baltimore, Maryland, which in 1919 was taken over by the Red Cross and in 1922 by the Rehabilitation Division of the Veterans Bureau under the name of Evergreen School for the Blind. In following the example of St. Dunstan (in England), it was not only medically but also rehabilitation orient- ed. (Lowenfeld, 1975, p. 150)

World War II produced many more blinded veterans, which led to a significant increase for funding rehabilitation centers, and in 1948, the Veterans Administration assumed a leadership role in providing such services.

THE SOCIAL CONTEXT OF AGENCY DEVELOPMENT

The decade preceding World War II saw major increases in federal funding and national support for several different programs. The Randolph-Shepard Act of 1936 authorized the vending stand program, which is funded by both federal and state money and a percentage of vendor sales. Blind people were given first choice in the procurement of vending stands on federal properties. Through state business enterprise programs, vendors were provided training and assisted in acquiring equipment. In doing so, the United States followed a successful Canadian program begun in 1920. As the program unfolded, most states followed the federal precedent that vending stands also be located on state-owned properties. Several amendments to the Act led to rapid expansion from 1,599 stands in 1954 to more than 2,242 in 1964. By 1996, there were more than 3,500 vending stands. This program now provides one of the largest sources of employment for blind people in the United States.

The National Industries for the Blind was launched in 1938 through the leadership and interest of Robert Irwin of the American Foundation for the Blind (Lowenfeld 1975, p. 157). This organization coordinated the procurement of materials, monitored the quality of products, and followed government orders to participating workshops. Workshops expanded output and made a significant contribution to the national war production effort during World War II.

> In 1973, eighty-three agencies in thirty-five states were associated with The National Industries for the Blind. Their sales amounted to $65,142,072, of which $29,865,935 were sales to the government and $35,409,602 to private industries for light manufacture and assembly contracts. These workshops employed 4,700 blind workers of whom 1,987 had additional handicaps. (Lowenfeld, 1975, p. 158)

By 1993, workshops associated with NIB had sales totaling $316,900,000. The NIB also maintains a research facility which develops new products and new production techniques. A percentage of workshop sales provide most of the support for the national program.

In 1935, the United States became the last Western industrial nation to develop a national Social Security system. One of its first provisions included grants to the states to provide several categories of aid to the blind, dependent, and the economically qualified elderly (Lowenfeld, 1975, p. 298). Title 10 provided federal funds for programs for blind people. "Retrospectively, it is interesting that among the amendments suggested by Robert B. Irwin, then Executive Director of the American Foundation for the Blind, was one to set aside funds to promote state activities in the field of care and rehabilitation of the blind," (p. 299).

Although created primarily for those who educated and provided services, during the 1930s, the American Foundation for the Blind (AFB) became the most effective national advocate for the cause of blind people. During this decade, the AFB also provided leadership and some of the resources for the Talking Book Program. Many of the first Talking Book machines were produced with resources from the Works Project Administration, another federal program to provide employment as part of the national effort to help during the Great Depression.

During this decade, organizations of blind people developed in several states. Within the advent of national policies and programs affecting blind people there was an obvious need, clearly seen by some blind people, for a strong voice to represent their interests in national policy debates. It was in this context that several states came together in Pennsylvania in 1940 and organized The National Federation of the Blind. Crucial to this development was the leadership of Jacobus tenBroek, who was elected the NFB's first president.

The federal and state public assistance programs were followed by the Supplemental Security Income of 1974. Although administered by the Social Security Administration, this program is paid for by government revenues. Recipients can earn limited amounts of money while still receiving SSI benefits, which are a significant source of support for many low income blind people in the United States today.

In fewer than 70 years the United States has witnessed an enormous proliferation of agencies offering services to blind people. These include sheltered workshops, schools, private agencies, rehabilitation centers and a wide array of programs provided by state agencies. Robert Scott has described three social conditions which favored the rapid expansion of these agencies: (1) The country was increasingly urbanized, which led to the creation of traffic and safety hazards for blind pedestrians. In rural areas, people were better known to each other and most felt a responsibility for the less fortunate, but "[i]n cities, the vast number of people of extrinsic relationships precluded individual responsibility for the plight of others. Individual responsibility was replaced by welfare services" (1969, p. 125). Blindness occurs infrequently in populations, but large urban areas created a social environment with relatively large numbers of blind people. For the first time, agencies brought together, educated, and trained them, a concept considered revolutionary in its day. (2) With assembly line industrial production, complicated tasks became more repetitive, permitting increased opportunities of employment for blind people. (3) The nuclear family became more common. Housing space was less available and more expensive and industrial work could not support an extended family. Wage earners frequently needed to relocate in the pursuit of employment opportunities.

> The extra cost involved in caring for a blind child, coupled with the fact that blind children remain dependent upon their families for longer periods of time than sighted children, absorb large sums of money that might otherwise be spent educating other children or purchasing the material goods that are the evidence of improved social standing. (p. 127)

The three conditions provided an environment in which agencies could solicit public support because they were offering services and activities which taught blind people the skills necessary for urban life. Employment in workshops, recreational opportunities for children and almost everything else that would keep blind people out of harm's way and make them less of a burden on their families suddenly became available.

WORKERS FOR THE BLIND

The proliferation of agencies and enhanced funding coming from state and government sources resulted in a steady increase in the number of workers providing services to blind people. Over the past fifty years, task specialization has become more common and the workers now make claims that they are professionals. This process can be understood in terms of the economic privilege and power which results for those occupational groups to whom the wider society accords professional status. "As professionalizing occupations move to create and affirm collective worth, one of the incentives for participation, as well as one of the major goals of the movement, is to secure support for individual dignity and individual careers" (Larson, 1977, p. 157).

When we review the growth of occupations which merged into the groups that currently claim professional status, we find conflicts which have resulted from several aspects of this process. By 1910, employment in the field of working with blind people was dominated by two organizations: the American Association of Instructors of the Blind (AAIB) and the American Association of Workers for the Blind (AAWB). The AAIB, founded in 1871, was primarily comprised of educators of the blind. The AAWB, founded in 1905, was a more broadly-based organization and included more blind workers. The agenda at the 1905 meeting of the AAWB included industrial education, employment, standardization of a tactual reading system, the welfare of elderly blind persons, boarding homes and other housing arrangements for blind adults, nurseries for blind babies and home teaching services for adults (Koestler, 1976).

The AAIB and AAWB had overlapping memberships and conducted separate biennial conventions in alternate years. In 1921, conferees from both conventions established the American Foundation for the Blind (Vaughan, 1993, p. 181).

This new organization was to fulfill the hope "that there should be in work for the blind some kind of General Foundation Representative of and responsive to every important phase or branch of the profession" (Koestler, 1976, p. 19). The American Foundation for the Blind (AFB), through successful fund raising efforts including those of Helen Keller, became a significant resource for the developing professions in work with the blind. The AFB continually sponsored national conferences on emerging topics of professional interest: for example, educational standards for home visitors and standards in the area of orientation and mobility. It also provided leadership and funding, in cooperation with the federal government, for the development and wide dissemination of the Talking Book Program.

Robert Irwin (1883-1951) became blind at age six, received a Masters degree from Harvard University, and became an influential leader in the AFB's early years. He and the AFB continually argued that specialized rehabilitation and education services were needed by blind people. This was one area in the United States upon which blind people and those who provide services have always been in agreement.

Many blind people, particularly the young and those incurring blindness in early or mid life, now confront a wide array of agencies and organizations involved in the rehabilitation and education process. These include schools for the blind, private agencies, sheltered workshops, professional organizations of specialized workers, state agencies, university training centers, and the accumulated state and national laws and policies. Most of these are new cultural creations in the United States and, in most cases, were influenced by earlier ideas and examples from Europe. The components of this system are all interdependent. Because the work is quite specialized, employment opportunities outside the system are limited. One either moves up in an agency or circulates within other parts of the system. The various parts of the system represent a considerable economic resource which the leadership attempts to expand and control. In general, professionals think they know more than anyone else about their fields of expertise. In work for the blind the professional leaders in the various areas usually think they should define "best practice" and what is good for blind people. Increasing numbers of blind people work within the

system and frequently view themselves in ways the profession sees as
appropriate. However, a significant number, both sighted and blind,
occasionally raise issues concerning the suitability of program efforts
for training or educating blind people to live independently in the
wider society. More than twenty years ago Lowenfeld observed:

> [T]here is no doubt that at one time in the history of the social status of the
> blind, agencies fulfilled an important function and have done much good for
> many blind people. Our question is whether agencies have advanced or
> obstructed integration. To this, the answer can only be that as a social force, the
> agencies have with few exceptions strongly tended toward paternalism and
> segregation, and neglected the potential that they have for serving as agents for
> integration. (1975, p. 292)

THE ORGANIZED BLIND

As mentioned above, urbanization resulted in increased numbers of
blind people living near each other and sometimes being brought
together in agency programs, workshops, schools, and so on. This was
accompanied by gradual improvement in the educational level of
most blind people and the development of autonomous organizations.
These include the National Federation of the Blind (NFB), founded in
1940, The Blind Veterans Association, founded at the end of World
War II; and the American Council of the Blind (ACB), founded in
1961. Of these, the NFB is the largest. It was established by a nationally prominent educator and legal scholar, Jacobus tenBroek. Seven
different states already had organizations of blind people; however,
under the leadership of Jacobus tenBroek, the NFB spread rapidly
throughout the United States.

Beginning in 1935, there was a nationwide federal government
response to economic problems linked to The Great Depression.
Some of the new policies related to blindness and this situation called
for a nationwide organization of blind people to respond to political
developments in the nation's capital. The motto of the new organization was "Security, Opportunity, Equality," and these goals are pursued through a wide variety of means including education of the general public and working to improve the cause of the blind through
state and national legislation. The NFB has directly confronted agencies over issues of exploitation and the custodial treatment of blind

people; direct picketing and litigation have been used (Vaughan 1997, pp. 171-198). This organization maintains that blind people should be involved in decisions affecting their lives. It also insists that the individuals best qualified to represent blind people are those designated by the democratically elected leadership of its state and national agencies. Obviously, all blind people do not belong to the NFB, just as all citizens do not participate in political parties that provide the leadership which governs the United States. However, self- appointed blind people represent only themselves, and they have sometimes been co-opted by agencies to lend an aura of legitimacy. The conflict has been greatest between the NFB and agencies or professions over issues of representation, exploitation, and control. During its first two decades, no issue received more attention than the exploitation of blind workers in sheltered workshops.

During the past 25 years, the issue of professional domination and the integrity of the evaluation process has produced intense conflict between the NFB and the National Accreditation Council for Agencies Serving the Blind and Visually Handicapped (NAC). The NFB has continually criticized and picketed the annual meetings of NAC. I have described this conflict in detail in my 1997 article, "Why Accreditation Failed Agencies Serving the Blind and Visually Impaired," published in the *Journal of Rehabilitation* (Vaughan, 1997). There have been additional fights over control or licensing of rehabilitation teachers. For example, the NFB has long argued that there is no great mystery to cane travel and that a blind person can teach it as well as anyone else. However, the dominant professional organization, the Association for the Education and Rehabilitation of the Blind and Visually Impaired (AER), has insisted on licensing only sighted mobility instructors. This organization is currently looking for "functional alternatives" as a way to get around this issue.

The NFB has an active program to place blind people in suitable jobs in the wider labor market. Three new residential rehabilitation centers are the Colorado Center for the Blind in Denver; B.L.I.N.D., Inc. (Blind Learning in New Dimensions) in Minneapolis; and the Louisiana Center for the Blind in Ruston. Almost all teachers in these agencies are blind and had to have worked in competitive employment before being deemed acceptable as rehabilitation teachers. Each center has a low student/teacher ratio and every aspect of the program stresses independent living and self-determination. These organizations have been remarkably successful in sending their students to higher education, competitive employment, and independent living (Vaughan, 1993, pp. 203-228).

At its National Center for the Blind in Baltimore, the NFB has developed technology to evaluate new programs that may be useful to blind people. Much money has been ill-spent because blind people themselves, those who would use the proposed new tools, were not involved in the early stages of development. As we near the twenty-first century it is impossible to overstate the potential of new technology for blind people. "However, technological advances, especially in translation of print and other visual information into sound, suggest that the history of blindness has entered a whole new era" (Safford and Safford, 1996, p. 152).

Perhaps the most important contribution of the NFB to the lives of blind people in the United States and in many other countries is its monthly publication, *The Braille Monitor*. This journal publishes articles on new developments in every area influencing the lives of blind people. It is made available in Braille, audio cassettes, and print, and currently has a monthly circulation of more than 29,000. The NFB also publishes another journal, *Future Reflections*, which is directed toward the parents and educators of blind children. Both journals are available through the National Federation of the Blind, 1800 Johnson Street, Baltimore, Maryland 21230, or through its web page address: http://www.nfb.org. A new publication was launched in 1986, *The Voice of the Diabetic*, published by The Diabetes Network of the National Foundation of the Blind, which is aimed at issues related to diabetes and blindness. Its distribution now exceeds 195,000 quarterly.

RECENT TRENDS IN THE EDUCATION OF BLIND CHILDREN

A major trend in special education has been the efforts to more fully integrate children with disabilities into the regular educational system. This has been a gradual process over the past quarter century, beginning with mainstreaming some children with mostly mild disabilities into regular classrooms for some portion of the day and moving toward the full inclusion of all children with disabilities for all of the day. This trend parallels and supports societal efforts to move toward greater acceptance of persons with disabilities and their fuller participation in all aspects of society. As mentioned above, as early as the mid-nineteenth century, Howe argued for having blind students remain at home and attend neighborhood schools as long as possible. More recently we have seen that Lowenfeld has expressed concern about how agencies have tended to obstruct integration of blind people into the full society.

Although the civil rights movement of the 1960s began with efforts to end discrimination against African-Americans, its arguments and advocacy efforts soon spread to other groups that were experiencing discrimination, including people with disabilities. Some children with severe disabilities, considered not "educable," were totally excluded from public schools. Minority groups were overrepresented in special education, particularly those of children labeled as having mild mental retardation. The concern was that these were often inappropriate placements, a subtle form of discrimination.

It was in this climate that The Education for All Handicapped Children Act of 1975 (PL 92-142) was enacted. It stated that all children were entitled to a free, appropriate education in the "least restrictive environment" and that families, for example those having a blind child, had to be involved in placement decisions. In 1990, this landmark legislation was updated and renamed the Individuals with Disabilities Education Act (IDEA). Other legislation has extended services to very young children, from birth to five years of age. The 1990 Americans With Disabilities Act, while dealing more with employment and accessibility issues than education, reflected the national commitment toward changing policies and attitudes toward the disabled. These federal laws have made inclusionary efforts a national mandate.

A major provision of these laws is that a child has the right to be educated in a setting closest to that provided for all children. "Mainstreaming" is the term that came to be used for placing the child with disabilities in general educational settings. Many children with disabilities who previously had been taught exclusively in separate classrooms were placed in regular classrooms. Mainstreaming could range from full participation to such minimal integration as having lunch or physical education with typical peers. Primarily, children with moderate to mild disabilities were mainstreamed. The criteria often used was that the child could be taught with minimal assistance in the regular classroom. Special classrooms continued for those with more severe disabilities.

During the 1980s the proponents of the Regular Education Initiative (REI) called for major changes in special education and mainstreaming as it was generally being practiced. Some went so far as to call for the merger of regular and special education and the elimination of the current dual system. One group of advocates were those concerned about children with learning disabilities, behavior disorders, and mild to moderate mental retardation–often called the "high-incidence" group of disabilities. Another group of advocates came from those concerned about children with severe disabilities (Kauffman and Hallaton, 1995). Neither of these groups included those concerned about blind children's education.

Advocacy for inclusive schools has become the focus of reform in the 1990s. The most vocal group has been from the second group of REI supporters, families of children with severe disabilities. TASH (The Association of Persons with Severe Handicaps) has pushed strongly for inclusion of children with severe disabilities who had generally not been part of earlier mainstreaming efforts. Full inclusion differs from mainstreaming in that all children, regardless of the severity or type of disability, are to be part of regular classrooms. Instead of "pull out" programs, all special services should be provided in the regular classroom and ideally by the regular teacher. Inclusion is for all children all of the time. They do not need to earn the right to be in the regular classroom nor is the amount of adaption a criterion for admission.

Most schools intend to provide a continuum of services for children with disabilities. They provide a range of options in the type of services offered and vary in the degree of classroom integration. At one end of this continuum are residential schools for blind students which are totally separate from the regular school setting. As discussed above, this has traditionally been the most widely practiced choice for blind children in the United States. In the self-contained classroom, children are in the same building as their peers but are in a class containing only other special education children. "Pull out" programs consist of mainstreaming children, then removing them for part of the day for special services, such as Braille or mobility training. "Reverse mainstreaming," a recent trend particularly with young children, is bringing typical peers into a special education classroom. This provides the desired peer modeling and social interaction. At the far end of the continuum is the full inclusion option. This means that the children receive services needed within the regular classroom and that specialists serve as consultants to the regular teacher or do direct intervention within the classroom.

Full inclusion is a controversial issue among both regular and special educators. Advocates of inclusion take the position that it is the right of children to be educated with their peers; they do not have to prove that they can meet certain standards. They argue that rather than putting the responsibility upon children to fit into the existing system, it is the educational system's responsibility to make whatever changes needed to make inclusion effective. They want them included because being in a regular classroom is beneficial for the total development of children with disabilities. Having typical peers as models increases their language, academic, and social skills. It also teaches all children positive attitudes toward those with disabilities–acceptance of differences and recognition that all have a right to full participation. Belonging to a classroom community and becoming an accepted and valued member of the group is thought to foster greater self-acceptance and self-esteem in children with disabilities.

However, difficulties arise in putting these principles into practice. A major concern is "dumping"–putting children with disabilities into regular classrooms without the reeducation of the regular teachers and without the support services needed. Too often such services are not adequately provided. Teachers feel overwhelmed by the additional responsibility and time involved and are sometimes unable to provide a good educational experience. For example, a blind child may receive very limited mobility training and Braille instruction if the regular teacher is not able to help the child utilize and advance in these very specialized skills. Even the special educator often has a very general orientation toward such blindness skills. One result has been that illiteracy among blind children is on the increase. Braille literacy laws have been passed in most states, but compliance is spotty at best. Often, instead of emphasizing Braille, the tendency is to try to get children to use whatever residual vision they have to read large print. This may be easier for the teacher, but not in the long-term best interest of the child.

EDUCATING DACIA

In the United States for the past several decades, Vocational Rehabilitation has received the greatest share of funding. Due to the aging of the population, many older people are experiencing visual loss for the first time and do benefit from services which promote independent living. As this chapter has illustrated, there has long been controversy over the best way to educate blind children. Consumer literature has frequently documented the difficulty parents have encountered in obtaining a desirable educational opportunity.

In my city, Columbia, Missouri, I am acquainted with a family which, to me, exemplifies how a family should involve itself in the education of a blind child. They modestly refer to their daughter as "average." I see her frequently and am convinced she is a well-adjusted and above- average thirteen year old. I asked her father, Lawrence Luck, to describe their experience in obtaining an education for their daughter which will maximize the various ways her life will be productive:

> Our daughter Dacia was born in March 1984, approximately three months early. When Dacia was about three months old, the hospital called to say the eye doctor had examined her. The physician informed us that Dacia had a high degree of retinal detachment in both eyes. We took Dacia from our home in Missouri to a specialized hospital in Memphis where she had surgery on both eyes before she was one year old, but the surgeries did not restore her sight.
>
> We were beginning to face the fact that our daughter would be blind for her entire life. As parents, one of our first concerns was fear and sympathy for our daughter. When Dacia was eighteen months old, the Rehabilitation Services Department of Missouri and the early childhood educators from our school district began home visits to establish a learning program for Dacia. School district educators informed us that some of Dacia's delays might be signs of mental retardation. Dacia has since proven that she is a normal child mentally. Jumping to the conclusion that blind children are retarded is common for early childhood educators in this country.
>
> Frequently, teachers feel sorry for blind kids and do not challenge them academically because of this pity. Professional educators can easily influence already concerned parents. This often negative influence can lead parents to feel that their blind children cannot lead a productive life in society.
>
> While Dacia was still in the preschool program, we met some members of a local organization of blind people. The group gave us some literature about blindness. Their literature informed us that the group worked hard to establish security, equality, and opportunity for the blind. A teacher from Rehab.

Services helped us get a subscription to their magazine for parents, *Future Reflections.* We began to attend local monthly meetings of the National Federation of the Blind (NFB). In a workshop sponsored by the NFB, we learned about Braille, IEPs and the education requirements in our country.

This workshop helped us gain hope that our daughter could live a very productive life and understand what goals to set for our child. Without the help of the NFB, I am sure we would have believed the school districts initial assessment of our daughter's mental status and their predictions about her limited ability to function in society.

Members of the NFB have helped Dacia and countless other blind individuals in many other ways. They have successfully convinced legislators in many states to set up Braille education bills that require public school districts to teach Braille to all children who need it. Dacia has also received some private Braille instruction from several members of the NFB. The NFB has worked hard to educate others that blindness is just a nuisance. The NFB also works hard to educate employers that blind people can be productive employees. Each year many blind people receive academic scholarships from the NFB so they may achieve their career dreams. Maybe, Dacia will someday receive one of these scholarships.

We are very proud to be a part of the NFB. Today our daughter reads and writes Braille very well. She is a successful student in the normal sixth grade curriculum. Although it took a lot of time to work things out, for the last few years she has been able to receive her school assignments in Braille at the same time that other students receive theirs. I would conclude by saying that Dacia can probably achieve her career goal of becoming a school teacher because of her hard work and the advocacy efforts of the NFB.

THE IMPORTANCE OF BRAILLE LITERACY

Technology and other aspects of our culture are changing so rapidly that education, including life-long education, is essential. Literacy is basic to quality education. However, literacy among blind people has been declining. This situation has been a major concern of many blind people, including the nation's largest advocacy group. Mr. Marc Maurer, an attorney and current President of the National Federation of the Blind, wrote the following statement for this chapter:

It is reported by the American Printing House for the Blind that the current literacy rate for blind school-age students has declined to approximately 9%. This is much lower than the literacy rate was for blind students decades ago.

At the same time, it has been estimated that as many as 85% of those who are blind and knowledgeable in the reading and writing of Braille are competitively employed. These two statistics suggest that Braille is important for the blind to achieve employment and to gain success in other areas, and that the teaching of Braille is on the decline. Unless the trend is reversed, long-term employment possibilities for blind people appear to be dismal.

A number of factors contribute to the crisis in Braille. Specialized teaching for the blind was from the middle of the nineteenth century to the middle of the twentieth century conducted almost exclusively at schools for the blind. At these residential settings, it was possible to concentrate resources so that blind students had the equipment and materials available to them that were specially adapted for teaching the blind students. Braille writers, Braille slates & styluses, Braille textbooks, Braille maps, white canes, and some other specialized equipment were maintained at the school. Because blindness occurs infrequently, schools not specially set aside for teaching the blind could not maintain the equipment and supplies. In addition, the specialized knowledge and skill required for teaching classes in Braille and cane travel was not possessed by teachers in the ordinary classroom.

In the late 1940's and throughout the 1950's, the number of blind children being born increased significantly. This put an intolerable burden on schools for the blind. By the late 1960's, there was an effort to offer education to blind students in the regular public schools. In 1974, the Education for Handicapped Children Act (now the Individuals with Disabilities Education Act--IDEA) was adopted. This law said that a free, appropriate public education would be available to all handicapped children. The effort to provide education to the handicapped in the regular public school setting became known as "mainstreaming."

Blind students found themselves being sent to the regular public schools. The argument was made that this would be beneficial because blind students learned alongside their sighted peers. It was felt that the socialization of the blind within the larger community would be of considerable benefit, and that a higher standard of education than was maintained in the school for the blind would be available then in the public school. Special teachers of the blind were expected to give lessons in blindness-related skills such as the use of Braille and the use of the white cane for travel. However, the substantial number of texts and other materials in Braille could not be kept at the school because the concentration of resources would cost too much. Furthermore, the school system did not have the money to hire specialized teachers for each blind student in each school. Not only were the funds not available to provide the teaching staff and the materials, but also administering the program which could make such resources available on only an intermittent basis in every single school system was simply impossible. Nevertheless, the law required education for blind children to be provided in the ordinary public school. This requirement removed the student population from the school for the blind and d i s - persed it throughout the public school system. The result is that education at the school for the blind is provided only to students with such limited capacity that the public schools cannot handle them. Unfortunately, blind students in the public schools frequently lack the skilled instructors and the materials that are essential for a top quality education. Hence, there is no adequate alternative.

There are, both in the public schools and at schools for the blind, efforts being made to alter this trend. At the present writing, there is a positive program of education for blind students being pursued at schools for the blind in Kentucky, Washington, Texas, and Indiana. It appears that there are also promising programs in South Carolina and Colorado. There are also some promising efforts in the public school systems. At one point Dr. Frederic K. Schroeder (who is currently serving as Commissioner of the Rehabilitation Services Administration) created an educational program for the blind in the Albuquerque public schools. This program achieved such dramatic results that it came to be a model for the nation.

Despite these positive instances in the educational system for the blind, the trends appear to be dismal. The National Federation of the Blind has recognized that there is a crisis in literacy for the blind. This national organization of blind people has instituted a nationwide campaign to improve literacy among blind students and to teach Braille to blind adults.

Braille bills drafted by the National Federation of the Blind, giving blind students the right to learn Braille in school, have been adopted by more than fifty percent of the states, and proposals for such legislation are actively being pursued in a number of others. In 1995, the NFB produced a video, "That the Blind May Read," a powerful summation of the failure of the educational system to teach blind people Braille. More than a thousand copies of this video have been distributed and it has appeared on television stations around the nation. In addition, we are working with the Association of American Publishers, the group of companies that produce primary and secondary school textbooks, to make more Braille texts available to students. The National Federation of the Blind is responsible for the production of more Braille than anybody else in the U.S. except the Library of Congress. We have created the International Braille and Technology Center, which houses   at least one of every Braille printer built anywhere in world. This facility is a laboratory for experimentation and comparison purposes for all technologies that produce Braille. We conduct classes to teach educators and rehabilitation professions the use of Braille-producing technology. We are supporting research into educational methods and techniques for teaching Braille both within the National Federation of the Blind and through the International Braille Research Center. We have supported and are distributing textbooks written by several different authors on the subject of teaching Braille. We are stimulating the teaching of Braille in towns and cities throughout the nation through community-based, self-help Braille discussion groups. We are conducting formal classes in Braille education through rehabilitation and adjustment centers in Minnesota, Colorado and Louisiana. We have and are distributing reference books in Braille, we have encouraged the production and distribution of children's books in Braille, and we conduct for blind youth an annual "Braille

Readers Are Leaders" contest which includes ceremonial presentation to the winners and cash prizes.

Professionals and consumers consistently agree that blind people must receive the requisite skills for independent living and self-determination. One of the dilemmas of the current educational approach is how to provide specialized educational services to blind children in "mainstream" or "full-inclusion" classrooms. Illiteracy has been on the increase because there are too few teachers with Braille skills and positive attitudes with regard to the use of Braille and the potential of blind students.

Another major concern is that the desired social integration does not occur. Just putting children with disabilities in a regular classroom does not guarantee positive social integration. Some children with disabilities may have a difficult time meeting the behavioral and academic expectations of a regular classroom. They may experience lack of acceptance by their peers, leading to isolation and a sense of rejection. Also of concern is the lack of successful blind role models. In schools for the blind, children work intensively with successful blind adults and peers. These positive role models can encourage them to strive for similar competencies and achievements. In a regular school setting blind children may have no experiences with blind adults or even other blind children.

In order to overcome these very real difficulties without foregoing the benefits of inclusion, many educators are recognizing the need for innovative approaches that challenge the traditional organizational structure and educational philosophies. Whether one goes so far as to argue for the blending of regular and special education into one totally unified system, most agree that a collaborative, interdisciplinary approach is essential. This means that regular and special educators, plus other specialists, should collaborate and jointly deliver needed services. Special educators provide both consultation for the regular teacher and direct intervention in the classroom. The ideal is that the special and regular teachers jointly share the planning and teaching for all children in the classroom. Special and regular education have in the past often differed in assumptions about how children learn and the type of teaching strategies to be used. These need to be reexamined and efforts made toward synthesizing differences and creating new approaches. Many believe such an overhaul is in the best interest of all children, not just those with disabilities.

The movement away from teacher-directed and whole class instruction to more child-initiated and peer group learning are changes that allow greater adaptation for children with disabilities. Strategies that allow for greater diversity of abilities and learning styles are evident in such recent trends as multi-age classrooms, cooperative learning groups, and the whole language approach for teaching reading and writing.

There is an increased recognition of the need to put significant effort into establishing a classroom climate that emphasizes cooperation, respect and responsibility for others, and positive attitudes toward differences. Teachers are actively seeking ways to facilitate social integration and build a sense of community. Such a classroom climate is beneficial to all children and especially important in helping a blind child feel an accepted part of the group. Families and schools need to provide opportunities for interaction with other children and adults with similar disabilities. Participating in such organizations as the National Federation of the Blind is one way to provide both valuable interaction and role models for blind children.

The Education for All Handicapped Children Act specifies that families should be participants in determining the educational goals and placement of their children. This is primarily accomplished through the Individual Education Plan (IEP), which must be completed annually for each child. In the past many families have been content with a relatively passive role. However, the growth of advocacy groups such as the National Federation of the Blind have been encouraging families to take a more assertive advocacy role for their children. Now they want more than information about decisions, they want to be centrally involved in the decision-making process. Across the nation, state affiliates of the NFB have become directly involved, sometimes through litigation, to bring recalcitrant school districts into compliance.

Part B and Part H of IDEA have extended the age at which children with disabilities should be served. There is widespread recognition of the benefits of early detection and intervention for disabilities, which make it even more important that a family-centered approach be used because this is the time when the families are the primary teachers and care givers for their children. It highlights the need for intervention efforts to focus on learning that takes place in their natural environment. It is through play, not isolated skills lessons, that young children learn best.

The implications for families with blind children are that they need to be actively involved in their child's education beginning at birth. They should take an active role in determining what goals and services are appropriate. They should not wait until the child is school age to begin such efforts as mobility training or literacy experiences. Efforts are specially needed during the early years when the families are the primary teachers of their children. Future Reflections, a journal mentioned above that focuses upon blind children, encourages families to be active in their child's education from a very early age. Many parents of blind children become regular participants in the NFB to learn from other parents and to expose their children to positive role models.

SUMMARY

The earliest programs for blind people in the United States were modeled after programs in Europe, and the education of blind children was the earliest concern. The failure of these students to find competitive employment gave impetus to the creation of sheltered workshops, which were soon separated from schools.

The first two decades of the twentieth century witnessed a rapid proliferation of private agencies, particularly in urban areas. Beginning shortly after World War I there was a continual expansion of federal and state funding to support education, rehabilitation, and welfare programs. The growth of private agencies and publicly supported programs led to a rapid increase in the number of workers. Following the lead of social welfare agencies, workers for the blind sought professional status and developed increased control over policy matters. The National Federation of the Blind, which became the largest and most influential organization of blind people, was born in 1940. Sometimes it has directly confronted agencies and groups of service providers within the profession over issues such as exploitation, representation and custodial treatment. The NFB has created a national center for the blind and has become one of the strongest forces for promoting the cause of blind people in the United States.

Chapter 5

BLINDNESS IN AFRICA

C. Edward Vaughan and Aubrey Webson

Africa is an extremely diverse continent, both culturally and geo-graphically. Even within individual countries there are usually many different languages, dialects, and ethnic groups with distinct cultural traditions. With only a few exceptions, most African countries have levels of economic development among the lowest in the world. In a single chapter, we can only discuss aspects of blindness that are widespread throughout Africa. Examples will come from countries with which we are most familiar, none of which lie north of the Sahara.

PREVENTION OF BLINDNESS

Prevention of blindness is an important goal, and such programs in Africa take many forms depending upon available medical technology and levels of economic development. For example, in most Western countries, the focus is on reducing accidents, early detection of diseases which can cause blindness if not corrected, and surgical intervention such as the removal of cataracts or repair of damaged retinas.

The poorest countries of the world have the highest prevalence of blindness. Most developing countries, including those in Africa, have rates of blindness ten times higher than those of more economically developed countries. As much as half of all blindness could be cured and a large percentage could be prevented. Cataract, trachoma, onchocerciasis, and xerophthalmia are among the top four causes of blindness in developing countries, with cataracts being responsible for

119

half of all cases. In Africa alone, it is estimated that there are about 3 million people blinded by cataracts. As life expectancy in Africa increases, so will the incidence of cataract blindness (Chiramabo, 1992). Cataracts can usually be cured with modern surgery. In Africa, south of the Sahara, the problem is growing because only one of ten cataracts is attended to through surgery.

Economic resources are seldom available from local sources to provide a broad public health approach to eradicate conditions causing blindness. The economic and social costs are compounded when the labor lost by unemployed blind people is considered. Efforts have been made to estimate the economic cost of blindness by taking into account the potential labor of a blind person over the work years of a lifetime. The International Non-Government Organization (INGO) Partnership Committee on Blindness Prevention, while making several plausible assumptions, has attempted to estimate these costs (see Table I). For a given geographic region their calculations include the average GNP per capita, the prevalence of blindness, the number of blind, the total working years lost due to blindness, and the loss per capita and total GNP due to blindness. The conclusion is dramatized by noting that the worldwide cost of blindness equals between one-sixth and one-fourth of the GNP of the United Kingdom. Thylefors summarizes these costs for regions with different levels of economic development. These calculations do not even include the cost of providing some type of "living" for unemployed blind people. Nevertheless, economic costs should not deflect attention from the needlessly diminished lives resulting from unnecessary social isolation.

The World Health Organization has provided leadership for a program in eleven West African countries to eliminate the small black fly that causes onchocerciasis or river blindness, the second leading infectious cause of blindness in the world after trachoma. Worldwide, more than 17 million people are infected by this parasite (*Los Angeles Times*, October 22, 1995, p. 4). It is estimated, for example, that approximately 4.5 million people have some form of this disease in the Republic of the Congo (formerly Zaire). "The disease starts insidiously. A female fly bites a human and unwittingly plants the parasites. Hard nodules of several worms grow under the skin, causing incessant itching. Victims scratch themselves raw. Millions of offspring like vermicelli, get into the bloodstream and worm themselves into the eyes"

(Duff-Brown, 1995 p. 5). Frequently, the result is blindness for the individual. Onchocerciasis is also a major cause of social and economic deterioration in several countries. Two major approaches show promise for greatly reducing and perhaps even eliminating this disease. Helicopters spray rivers where

Table 2. The Cost of Global Blindness.

Global Economic Division (a)	Low Income Economics	Middle Income Economics	High Income Economics	World Total
Population (millions) 1993(a)	3092	1596	812	5500
GNP per capita (USS) 1993 (a)	380	2480	23090	4420
Prevalence of blindness (%) (b)	0-8	0-5	0-3	0-7
Number of blind people(millions) (b)	Adults 24-5 Children 0-9	Adults 24-5 Children 0-3	Adults 9-5 Children 0-2	Adults 36-5 Children 1-4
Total working years lost due to blindness (c)	0-10 0-50	0-10 0-50	0-10 0-50	0-10 0-50
GNP per capita lost due to blindness (growth rate = 3% USS 1993 (d)	380-511 380-1666	2480-3333 2480-10872	23090-31031 23090-101224	4420-5940 4420-19377
Total GNP lost due to blindness (growth rate = 3%) USS 1993 (d)	9310-12520 342-1499	23560-31644 744-3262	57725-77578 4618-20245	161330-216810 6188-27128
Total GNP lost due to preventable or curable blindness (growth rate = 3% USS millions 1993 (f)	6983-9375 171-750	17670-23748 372-1631	43294-58184 2309-10122	120998-162608 3094-13564

(a) Data taken from the World Development Report 1995.[5]
(b) Data taken from Thylefors et al. 2
(c) This represents an average number of working years lost due to blindness for all causes and the actual number of years may be lower.
(d) Given the GNP per capita x$(1-03)^{0-10}$ x number of blind adults and GNP per capita x $(1-03)^{0-50}$ for childhood blindness.
(e) Given by GNP per capita x $(1-03)^{0-10}$ x number of blind adults and GNP per capita x $(1-03)^{0-10}$ x number of blind children.
(f) This column is obtained by multiplying column (e) by 0.75 the total cost of adult blindness and by 0.5 the total cost of childhood blindness.

conditions are favorable breeding grounds for the fly, killing the larvae and thus preventing the transmission of the parasite to humans. The second approach involves a new drug which is being contributed, without charge, by the Merck Pharmaceutical Company. "The recent development of a safe, effective drug, Ivermectin, capable of causing clinical improvement and decreasing the transmission of infection, has led to a new global strategy for controlling onchocerciasis based on yearly administration of Ivermectin to affected populations" (WHO, 1995).

Trachoma, the leading cause of blindness in this region, is a contagious infection of the cornea and conjunctiva. The bacterium causing this condition can be controlled or limited through enhanced hygiene. Where literacy rates are low, public health education is more difficult. Education through direct contact at the village level is the most promising educational approach.

If economic resources are available and social conditions are favorable for diffusing information, xerophthalmia can also be prevented. This disease is caused by a deficiency of Vitamin A and is characterized by the eye being dry and lusterless. It can be successfully improved through the use of Vitamin A and the dispersal of nutritional information. Cataracts are a large and growing source of blindness in most African countries.

> The backlog of cataract cases is still considerable and continues to increase whilst the cataract surgical rate remains unacceptably low. The reasons for this are multifactorial and include poor patient recruitment, high cost to the patient, sub-optimal use of existing personnel and quality of service which does not meet the expectations of patients. (Thylefors, 1997, p. 8)

One of the problems is the shortage of ophthalmologists. For example, Ghana has only 32 ophthalmologists, one per eight hundred thousand. Many other African countries have even fewer ophthalmologists per capita than Ghana.

Africa has had its share of civil conflicts which have resulted in war-related injuries, also contributing to high rates of blindness. In many cases, there is conflict between ethnic groups struggling for political domination in artificially structured governments created arbitrarily by colonial administrators. In addition to many of the countries affected by civil conflict, natural disasters such as droughts cause forced migration, frequently resulting in poor sanitary conditions. For many, survival is the most immediate concern.

The World Health Organization is launching Project 2000 in cooperation with major NGO's to heighten efforts to prevent and cure blindness because of the enormous increase anticipated in population and life span by the year 2020. Most of these countries have developed and are developing programs to prevent blindness, special education and rehabilitation programs to promote independent living, and employment opportunities. Most countries in Africa have developed organizations of blind people which have seen growth in membership, political influence, and leadership. In a great many cases, economic and technical support have been provided by more economically developed countries.

TRADITIONAL VIEWS

Africa, contrary to many outside stereotypes, is both ethnically and culturally quite diverse. Traditional folk cultures in many parts of Africa have popular beliefs about blindness and physical disabilities that observers in many parts of the world would recognize. There are beliefs which correspond to Western notions that parental sour grapes may put children's teeth on edge. Professor Nicholls of Howard University observed a tendency to reduce African ideas about disability to a few hackneyed scenarios in which disability is seen either as a result of witchcraft, for example, ill intent directed from a human agency by supernatural means, or as a form of divine retribution visited on a negligent individual for failing to observe a religion's code or for breaking a taboo (1993, p. 26). These traditional explanations certainly exist, but are often taken out of a larger, more positive context. The traditional stereotypes are frequently reinforced by outside reports about the condition of blind people in Africa. For example, in an October 22, 1995 article (Part A, p. 4), the *Los Angeles Times* describes a family in which most members have onchocerciasis. Two of the mother's sons died from the disease and another adult son is blind. She explains her blindness thus: "It was a sorcerer who caused this . . . I didn't do anything wrong; someone did this to me." She has isolated herself in her hut because "she does not want to be a burden."

She affirms that the devout Muslim villagers have treated her well. She and many like her have had no opportunity to learn the parasitic/disease cause of her blindness.

Nicholls comments further on the diversity of cultural beliefs about disability. Among the Ngwa Igbo, albinos and physically handicapped people are thought to have sinned in their previous lives. Concerning the Yoruba of Nigeria, many disabilities are perceived to be the work of wizards as punishment for offenses. For example, blindness is thought to be caused by black magic resulting from jealousy (1993, p. 26).

Nicholls demonstrates that there is wide diversity in the way disability is viewed in Africa. He describes an East African group in which the physically disabled are protected because their presence is thought to ensure the health of others. Children with physical disabilities in Benin are cherished because they are thought to be gifts of spirits which bring good luck. Nicholls also describes other instances in which tribal customs provide positive support and protection for people with disabilities. We share many of Professor Nicholls' opinions concerning positive features often overlooked in traditional societies.

> Instead of recognizing that traditional African ideologies contain real wisdom, negative views of traditional culture have prevailed and an idea promoted that African cultures are more "primitive" and "barbaric" than so-called "civilized" cultures. In recent years this bias has been changing and scholarly areas such as ethnoscience and ethnomedicine have emerged which look at traditional cultures as a source of valuable knowledge. In addition, there is now a body of opinion that suggests that traditional African societies are in many ways more "human" and more "humane" than modern industrial societies. (1993, p. 25)

Professor Nicholls provides extensive bibliographic references on topics related to ideas about health, the treatment of illness, and attitudes toward disability. He also names various sources describing the supportive nature of social relationships in most African villages. In addition, he cites a prominent French anthropologist, Jacques Maquet, who claims, "African societies . . . are much better than industrial societies at organizing human relationships so as to reduce tensions and anxieties" (1993, p. 25).

Within a given country, attitudes toward blindness among tribal groups can be quite diverse. In Ghana, for example, the tribal chief of the Ashanty was not to encounter a blind person. If he did, he had to go home and make a sacrifice to cleanse himself so that he broke no taboo. Another folk belief in Ghana was that encountering a blind person first thing in the morning was a bad omen for the whole day. In several African language groups within Ghana, words used for blindness or disabilities carry the meaning of sickness. The Akan is the largest tribal group in Ghana. Among the Ashanti, a tribe related to the Akan, the blind descendants of a tribal chief could not be successors, nor could a blind male be the head of a family.

On the positive side, in the northern districts of Ghana, the Fra Fra people view blindness in a positive light. In this tribe and others in the North, blind people are well integrated and regarded as normal. We could find no clear explanation for this, except perhaps that there were so many blind people in this district that they could not be ignored. In fact, blind people were chiefs, heads of households, and had no problem assuming their cultural duties. In these same tribes, blind women who had no contact with organizations of or for blind people were taught the ordinary customs and roles associated with being female. They became married, worked within the family, and farmed. They learned these things through traditional tribal resources, not from outside intervention programs.

In addition to changing images and attitudes through public education and awareness programs, successful blind people are changing cultural ideas about blindness. For example, in Ghana, one blind man is employed as a government attorney. Representing national government programs, he visits different tribal groups, sitting in the "house of chiefs" where he can hardly be ignored. Although he is blind, they interact with him in terms of equality, in spite of cultural traditions.

Prevention and treatment efforts may be more effective when they take advantage of the strengths of local cultural traditions. Folk medicine and ethnic healers should not be overlooked as resources. "It was noted that traditional healers have been accessible to rural Africa for centuries. It is recommended that through interaction, dialogue and education, the healers are informed on eye care delivery and their cooperation and collaboration be sought on eye care delivery and prevention of harmful practices particularly at the community level" (Thylefors, 1997, p. 9).

Regardless of the cultural strengths apparent in many African traditions, there are few economic opportunities for most blind people in most parts of the continent. For many, survival itself is difficult and begging is the only alternative. With limited economic resources, there are few education and rehabilitation opportunities. All over Africa different types of programs are being built on traditional cultural values to eradicate some of the common causes of blindness, to provide education and rehabilitation and to give African men and women more economic alternatives and fuller participation in society.

THE IMPORTANCE OF GENDER–SEXUAL RELATIONSHIPS BETWEEN THE BLIND AND THE SIGHTED

To sociologists, gender is in every society and culture a dimension of social inequality. Gender refers to the significance a society attaches to the differences between males and females. In some industrialized societies, gender relationships have been changing rapidly during this century. Traditional and less economically modernized societies are changing slowly and patriarchal patterns of domination are more evident. Sexuality is a dimension of our human condition and it is no less significant in the lives of blind people. William Rowland describes what he learned from surveys about what blind people considered most important for enjoyment of life. Family comes first. "And when people talk about family life they refer to all aspects and to all stages–to being a child, a brother or sister, to getting married and having children, and to growing old among your own people" (1993, p. 17). Rowland reports that another expressed need is for the experience of sex itself, a frequent topic of conversation among blind people and openly talked about in discussion groups (1993, p. 17). In spite of cultural differences, blind people around the world share with other people interests in stable family relationships and in intimacy. However, traditional, deeply ingrained cultural ideas about gender relationships, the proper role relationships ascribed to men and women, can greatly complicate the lives of blind people, particularly those of women living in male dominated societies.

Nayinda Sentumbwe is an anthropologist, a man who grew up in Uganda and who also happens to be blind. He has analyzed the cultural conditions which prevent many blind women from experiencing traditional family relationships. In several ethnic groups within

Uganda, words used to describe blindness convey the meaning of helplessness. "Because of the vulnerable state people imagine blind people to be in, loss of sight is for most Ugandans, therefore, perceived to be the most disabling of all physiological disabilities" (Sentumbwe, 1993, pp. 52-53). Blind people are made painfully aware of these attitudes when they are denied culturally valued and culturally prescribed roles, and they may be partially or totally denied access to desired activities or relationships. Sentumbwe analyzes the prospects of blind women for marriage. In Uganda, males have better marital prospects than females. In many cultures, blind women are more likely to marry blind men than the reverse. Sentumbwe cites research from Norway which shows that blind women are more likely to marry blind men, while blind men are more likely to marry sighted women (p. 54). In Uganda, blind women do have relationships with blind men, but these are usually casual. The main condition which restricts opportunities for blind women is traditional gender roles. In Uganda, marriage is an affair between two families. Close kin and other relatives are traditionally called in to approve a prospective spouse, particularly when the spouse is female. In-laws expect to receive various services from the new family members. "Like most women in other societies, once married, the Ugandan woman traditionally fulfills most household roles: mother, hostess, house and homestead-keeper, provider of meals, provider of homegrown food, etc." (Sentumbwe, 1993, p. 54). She is also supposed to keep good relations with the relatives and neighbors. Weddings, funerals, and other important ceremonial occasions usually involve clear-cut expectations for women. If these tasks are not well performed, even the husband can be criticized for selecting an undesirable wife. In this context, it is not difficult to understand why men see blind women as candidates for casual sexual contact, but not for marriage partners.

It is difficult for blind girls to learn requisite social skills. In order to be protective or perhaps because they expect little,

> The parents of blind girls, particularly the mothers, have a negative attitude toward their daughters. Because of this, they fail to give their blind daughters an informal education at home in such things as daily cooking, washing, keeping babies, and so on, skills which are necessary for the future of the blind girl who intends to get married. This problem, therefore, is extended into the womanhood of a blind girl. (Mpirirwe and Diri-Baba, 1997, p. 162)

Aubrey Webson (1997) has observed on his frequent trips to most countries in Africa that blind women have acquired the usual array of housekeeping and homemaking skills. It is possible that Mpirirwe and Diri-Baba overstate the matter, or perhaps blind girls learn these skills in ways other than in the usual mother-daughter relationships.

The educational system itself heavily favors men. "In many co edu-cational institutions, where more residential facilities are allocated to the male at the expense of the female, this trend is not different in either special schools or rehabilitation centers" (Fefoame, 1996, p. 167). Patriarchism exists worldwide and is a distinct feature through-out Africa. In Fefoame's Ghana, "an African woman is regarded basi-cally as a vehicle of procreation while the man allots himself the right of production and decision making. As decision makers, they make sure everything favors them. This trend of affairs was accepted and perpetuated by women over the years" (1996, p. 166).

Many people in some traditional ethnic groups within Uganda regard blind women with complete disdain. They think that blind women can not measure up in traditional homemaking, love making, dancing, and so on. They can not inherit property or anything else, nor be paid her dowry. Thus, some traditional beliefs and social cul-tural practices stand in the way of blind women leading normal lives or even benefiting from rehabilitation programs. To escape these con-straints, such women must make great sacrifices by living away from their families and traditional communities (Mpirirwe and Diri-Baba, 1997). In their 1996 presentation to the first African Forum on Rehabilitation (April 22, 1996 Accra, Ghana), Mpirirwe and Diri-Baba paint a bleak picture for young, Ugandan blind women. "First of all, very few blind girls go to school. Secondly, those who do go drop out as a result of rampant pregnancy caused by both sighted and blind men. Thirdly, government and other nongovernmental organizations (NGOs), do not consider blind girls for sponsorship" (p. 163).

Despite the problems mentioned above, there are now 15 blind women employed as teachers in Uganda. More than 50 blind women have been made aware of the negative attitudes they must overcome, and some have become involved in self-help projects. Blind women now come together to discuss their mutual concerns through the Ugandan National Association of the Blind and are now participating in leadership development seminars (Mpirirwe & Diri-Baba, 1997, p. 164).

INTERNATIONAL COOPERATION

In many parts of the world, government resources are too meager to support adequate levels of programs for education and rehabilitation. Even when funds are available, other claims may win the political battle over resources, and blindness may be viewed as far less important on the agenda for national economic development. Only in 1996 did the United Nations conduct its first "world summit" on social development, a belated recognition that this arena of life has always taken a back seat to economic issues. In recent decades there have been growing levels of cooperation among government, international non-government, and private organizations with concerns about blindness. Most countries in Africa, to varying degrees, have benefitted from these shared resources.

The United Nations, the United Nations Development Program (UNDP), UNICEF, the World Health Organization, the World Bank, the International Monetary Fund, and the International Labor Organization have each worked through existing government structures to promote economic and social development in Africa. Frequently, there are attempts to coordinate these efforts with international nongovernment organizations and indigenous organizations within host countries. As noted in Chapter 2, these international organizations frequently promote generic approaches to rehabilitation practices. This is a serious problem because most organizations of blind people and those who provide them education and rehabilitation agree that the most effective programs are those specializing in services required for independent living, literacy, and vocational training.

International cooperation also occurs through nongovernment organizations. In 1990, the International Development Project (IDP) was launched under the auspices of the World Blind Union. Initially, the major international programs involved included: Sight Savers International (United Kingdom), the Hilton/Perkins International Programme based at the Perkins School for the Blind, (U.S.), and the Canadian National Institute for the Blind (CNIB), and several countries in Africa are participating. Frequently, additional organizations outside Africa share the costs and will meet the expenses of local operation. One of the largest international contributors to programs worldwide is the German-based, Christoffel Blindenmission.

PAN-AFRICAN COOPERATION

If for no other reason, economic pressures have encouraged cooperation among African countries. We have already mentioned the
shortage of Braille material for adult readers: production is expensive
and, optimally, involves modern technology. For example, small countries such as The Gambia cannot, at this time, afford the necessary
equipment. Through Pan-African Cooperation, Braille could be published at one or two sites and made available throughout the continent.
College level instruction in matters related to rehabilitation could be
accomplished most effectively at one or two university sites, rather
than in many locations. Making books and magazines available on
cassettes through a Pan-African system of lending libraries would be
extremely important. Because of the traditions of aural learning and
the low levels of Braille literacy, recorded books would be a major
asset to education efforts and would also enrich the lives of enormous
numbers of blind people. Perhaps recorded books could be borrowed
from various European countries or from the Americas and be dupli-
cated and distributed from one or two sites. Ideally, books would be
recorded in Africa in order to reflect local linguistic practices. One
example of an African source is Tape Aids for the Blind of South
Africa.

Cooperation among countries already occurs in several different
ways. For example, in the 1960s and 70s some blind children from
Uganda attended school in Kenya. Many blind students and teachers
of the blind from Francophone West Africa attended school or training facilities in Tunis, while children and teachers from The Gambia
attended school in Ghana and or Sierra Leone. In the 1980s, the
Montford training college in Malawi became a major training institution for orientation and mobility specialists and for teachers from
throughout the Anglophobe region of Africa. Its programs were supported by many international nongovernment organizations, including Sight Savers of the U.K. and CBM of Germany.

In 1982, Sight Savers, working in collaboration with its partners in
East, Central, and Southern Africa, developed a computerized Braille
production unit in Kenya. The ABCD project was designed to produce Braille in support of education programs in countries in Southern
and East Africa. It produces master texts and has satellite units in

many of the cooperating countries, including Kenya, Uganda, Zimbabwe, and Botswana. Today it produces Braille in more than six African languages. To date, the Sight Savers approach through the ABCD project is the major effort made at deliberately designing a program aimed at a Pan-African answer to the problem of services for the blind on the continent.

In October 1987, the consumer movement, guided by the WBU began the establishment of regional unions among its members. Delegates came together in Tunis and held the first meeting or general assembly of the African Union of the Blind (AFUB). The Union held its second meeting in 1992 in Cairo, Egypt, and shortly afterward opened its secretariat in Nairobi, Kenya. The African Union of the Blind now involves more than thirty countries, and one of its main functions has been to foster the development of organizations of blind people in countries where such groups do not exist or are ineffective. The Union's cooperation is funded by the Norwegian Association of the Blind and Partially Sighted. In 1995, a WBU sponsored conference for blind women in Africa resulted in the formation of the AFUB Women's Committee. In 1996, at the Union's third general assembly (Nairobi, Kenya), Gertrude Fefoame of Ghana was elected first woman on its executive board when she was elected as Vice President.

As the demand for scarce international resources for social services continues to grow exponentially, blind people will continue to compete against those in need of short-term and immediate relief programs, such as those brought on by wars and natural disasters. These resources are also in demand for life-threatening diseases such as HIV, measles, malaria, and so on. Because crisis conditions nearly occur on a day-to-day basis, the needs of blind people and the disability movement in general are further pushed to the side. In the wake of this situation, blind people and their organizations must increase intraregional cooperation. To this end, the need for sharing expertise, both physical and human resources, and information are critical and will demand strategies that allow the blindness system to meet its own challenges from within. The response to this need will begin with blind persons and their organizations taking a Pan-African approach to the sharing of information, exchange of personnel, and the development of existing physical resource facilities. Such an approach will also provide African answers to African problems. The Africa Forum of April 1996 in Accra, Ghana, and subsequent regional meetings such as those of the ICEVI and the AFUB, began the process of intraregional sharing. However, many challenges remain.

At the beginning of this chapter, we noted the great diversity of cultures on the African continent, most of which have national boundaries set by former colonial administrators. In many ways, ethnic conflict is frequently related to these boundaries. Likewise, most rehabilitation programs have developed in the context of colonial arrangements; that is, former British colonies are more likely to benefit from international cooperative efforts associated with the British commonwealth, since relationships are strongest with the United Kingdom and Canada. In like manner, former French colonies are more likely to be associated with cooperative efforts from France. Several European countries which had minimal imperialist involvement in Africa, such as the Scandinavian countries, also provide economical and technical assistance to some countries.

Organized rehabilitation programs occur throughout Africa. This chapter focuses on countries in the Sub-Sahara region, particularly Uganda, Ghana, Zambia, South Africa, and The Gambia. The progress of many additional countries could be discussed further, but this would go beyond the scope of this chapter. For our purposes, we will next look at countries with relatively strong indigenous organizations of blind people.

THE GAMBIA

The Gambia is the smallest country on the continent of Africa and with 1.6 million residents, it is densely populated. The economic resources available to this country would permit minimum education and rehabilitation services for its blind citizens. The Gambia Organization for the Visually Impaired (GOVI) illustrates the kind of progress that can occur through international cooperation. The International Development Project has provided intensive leadership seminars for blind people in The Gambia. Founded in 1991, it is dedicated to the social and economic well being of its members.

GOVI was organized to reflect the following ideas:

1. Faint voices raised here and there are difficult to perceive, but when they unite, then they can be a force that will require attention;

2. Their liberation from the bonds imposed on them by a still ignorant world will progress slowly without their own active participation;

3. They live in an era where their needs go far beyond the simple provision of food, clothing and security by the family clan or village;

4. They cannot depend on hand outs from social welfare systems which are yet to keep even pace with developments.[1]

One of GOVI's main concerns is the education of children. Hence, Braille is taught at their resource center in Campama. After becoming literate in Braille, students take part in the regular school system. At the resource center at Campama, students are also taught independent living skills. Likewise, adults are taught skills for independence that lead to self-determination and are taught vocational skills appropriate to their interests or aptitudes. During the few years since its inception, GOVI has had several success stories. Four of their members are now involved in college studies in the United States; four others are rehabilitation teachers; seven are government employees and three are self employed.[2] GOVI has become the largest provider of services for the blind in The Gambia.

The GOVI's headquarters are 100 meters from Campama Primary School, the site of its resource center, at 41 Box Bar Road. It has ten affiliates in The Gambia and it supplies all blind Africans with knowledge, skills training, and information. Some of its projects include a multi-purpose center, orchards, vegetable gardens, sheep and goat farms, and a women's poultry project. "[These] free services which GOVI operates with assistance from foreign donors, subvention from The Gambia government and locally raised funds promotes the individuality and independence of all Gambian blind and visually impaired persons."[3]

The following is an account of one man's experience of blindness in mid-life. It illustrates the kind of resources that are only available through international cooperation. Mr. Lamin Siane held the rank of Captain in The Gambia Armed Forces when he was involved in a severe auto accident in 1993 (Siane, 1997).

---

1 These ideals are quoted from GOVI The Gateway for Information Knowledge & Vocational Training for All Blind and Visually Impaired Persons in The Gambia: Vision 2020, a newsletter circulated in June 1997, p.5.

2 IBID, p.6

3 IBID, p.7

FROM LOSS OF SIGHT TO REHABILITATION– ONE PERSON'S EXPERIENCE

Following a car crash which resulted in serious damage to the retinae and cornea in both of my eyes, I was evacuated from my home in The Gambia to Moorfields Hospital in London. Better services and equipment for opthamological surgery were available in London.

I underwent treatment in London a week after the accident in the same month of June 1993. The treating surgeon, Dr. Robert Cooling, then informed me that the loss of sight was going to be permanent, but that he was going to do his best to help me regain navigational vision. I did have that and while I was leaving hospital, he gave me letters of introduction to Sight Savers International and to the Head of Campama Resource Center (the School for the Blind in The Gambia). I got both letters delivered on my arrival back to The Gambia. I was then hospitalized locally for some three weeks during which I received follow-up care in the Eye-Ward of The Royal Victoria Hospital. During this period, I was visited by the Head of Campama Blind School. She was, on that occasion, accompanied by the Executive Secretary of The Gambia Organisation of the Visually Impaired.

. In September 1994, when I was finally declared permanently blind by a medical board, I returned to the Office of the President of The Gambia where I was employed prior to the mishap. I was asked to return to work.

At the work place I soon discovered that I had to dictate everything and everything had to be read to me. I then visited the blind organisation's headquarters to tell the people that I needed their services after all. I had earlier thought that I did not because I was confident and hopeful that the little sight I was gaining would have eventually enabled me to read and write. It did not and so I resorted to the only choice left.

I got registered at the school for the blind and applied for membership in the Organisation. As time went on, I learnt to read and write Braille and participated in other activities of the Organisation. I attended workshops, conferences, meetings, etc., in The Gambia and on one occasion in Ghana.

It was during these activities that I met Mr. Aubrey Webson, an IDP consultant who showed much concern about my particular situation. It was through him that I was admitted to Optima College in Pretoria, South Africa in October 1996. During my two months of Independence Training at Optima, I improved my skills in Braille and typing and further to do Word Perfect and also to use Braille and Speak. I practised daily living skills, orientation and mobility, as well as interacting with many blind and sighted persons who have trained and worked with the blind. I was also exposed to the South African larger society where the blind are treated almost as the sighted.

In addition to acquiring knowledge, I returned home with a lot of equipment such as a computer, Braille and Speak, a dictaphone and smaller items like a liquid level indicator. I got registered as a member of the Tape Aid for the Blind and do receive cassettes regularly.

I presently carry on with my job more easily and participate more actively in the affairs of The Gambia Organisation of the Visually Impaired (GOVI). Reading material that I receive from the Royal National Institute for the Blind (United Kingdom) is also of tremendous use in my rehabilitation.

UGANDA

The Uganda National Association of the Blind was formally organized in 1970. In its early years, the organization accomplished little and lacked clear objectives.

> With no programmes, the organization's main direct contribution to the membership was the distribution of white canes and writing slates whenever they were available. On occasion, the leaders attended international conferences, but no programmes were coordinated to disseminate information to the general membership. (Isiko, 1995, p. 36)

Local leadership among the blind had only a limited perspective on possible future developments. The civil strife occurring in Uganda during this period further weakened the UNAB. Nelson Isiko, the Secretary General of UNAB, described this earlier condition as a time of "hopelessness and despair" for most blind people. By 1987, the organization was in disarray. "In 1988 the government of Uganda stepped in, suspended the executive board and gave the responsibility of reorganizing the Association to the National Movement for the Disabled" (p. 36).

The UNAB began to reorganize itself and held an election in 1990. Subsequently, it became separate from the government sponsored programs for disabled people, and an effort was made to improve the organization by broadening the leadership base. The new leadership wanted to develop the capability to provide services to its members. At this time, the UNAB became involved with the Institutional Development Program. "Through this first exercise of management development training, the Board of UNAB for the first time was able to set an annual programme, and set targets by which it would be evaluated" (Isiko, 1995, p. 37). Subsequently, the general public began to take notice of the new vitality of the UNAB. Through a nationwide diffusion of the IDP program, more than 600 blind people became involved in leadership training programs.

> Specifically, more than seventy-five blind persons in Uganda have been exposed to direct training through the IDP in the following categories: holding effective meetings, leadership styles and methods, problem identification and problem solving, needs assessment, the structure of a membership organization and the role of its component parts, project formulation and proposal writing, budgeting and accounting at organizational and personal levels, communication as an effective means of administration, setting up viable projects, public relations and strategic planning, community participation, evaluation and monitoring, and probably most important of all, developing personal skills, gaining and sharing personal information for survival and function as a blind person in a developed society. (p. 37)

As a result, the UNAB has gained national respect and is participating in the nation's efforts at social and economic development. While independent, the UNAB has worked with other disability groups to obtain representation in the national legislative process. Also, the UNAB has contributed to numerous new projects, including rehabilitation and income generating ones. Several new units have been created for the education of blind children. Initiatives are now underway to provide service to the deaf blind. Recently, a program to educate the parents of blind children has been created. This program is based on the philosophy that parents are important educators and can be significant advocates for the needs of blind children. When the organization develops to the point that volunteers cannot provide necessary leadership to move to a new level of service delivery, some full-time workers will be required. "UNAB is undoubtedly a better and stronger organization because of the intervention of the IDP. Blind persons in Uganda have seen another way, and life once again has meaning" (Isiko, 1995, p. 38).

Blind people in Uganda have frequently worked in coalition with other disability groups. In fact, Uganda has become a model by involving disabled people in government affairs. " 'Society's attitudes toward people with disabilities are definitely changing in Africa,' said Seth Mpooya, deputy executive director of the National Union of Disabled People of Uganda. 'More of us have jobs. Our standard of living is higher. People see that we are as smart as anybody else' " (Buckley, 1997, p.14). These changes in attitudes have wrought extraordinary results in places such as Uganda, where at least five members of parliament are people with disabilities. Recently, the government appointed a disabled person as judge, which is believed to be unprecedented there (p.14).

In his recent book, *The Empowerment of the Blind* (1997), Aubrey Webson outlined the accomplishments of the Uganda National Association of the blind:

- Blind people in Uganda, for the first time, are influencing the development and delivery of services through their own organizations.
- Since 1990, the UNAB has been responsible for a 67 percent increase in the number of its branches.
- It now provides support for more than one thousand blind people, a 40 percent increase.
- It has established a national office in Kampala.
- It provides training for its personnel at all levels.
- The UNAB has established income-generating projects for several of its branches.
- It supports a special family rehabilitation and counseling program for blind women.
- It supports other advocates for the blind.
- It has been instrumental in tripling the number of blind children attending school.
- It works with a national support group for parents of blind children.
- It supports the development of a deaf-blind association that provides services for deaf-blind persons.
- It has increased by 40 percent the number of blind people involved in programs for the blind.
- It has reorganized its structure to include a cross section of blind people.
- It has organized local and international fund raising campaigns.
- It is developing local resources to help support many of its activities. (1997, p. 18)

GHANA

In the 1950s and 60s, the former Royal Commonwealth Society for the Blind (now Sight Savers), worked with national governments throughout former Anglophobe Africa to establish Society's for the Blind. The Ghana Society for the Blind was one of the first, and was established in the late 1950s. In Ghana, Uganda, Tanzania, and Kenya, through the RCSB, many rehabilitation centers were dedicated to the service of blind persons. The first president of Ghana, Dr. Kwame Nkrumah, dedicated several rehabilitation centers around the country to the training of blind persons. He made a strong national commitment toward providing services for blind people.

Currently, there are several agencies coordinating rehabilitation work for the blind in Ghana. The Ghana Society for the Blind (GSB) was the earliest agency to begin the provision of rehabilitation services to the blind in Ghana. GSB was formed in the 1950s. It was formerly a commonwealth member of the RCSB, now Sight Savers. The Ghana Association of the Blind, was founded by blind men who worked within the rehabilitation centers. These men formed the association in an attempt to give a voice to blind people in the development of services. With the support of the first president of Ghana, blind persons trained in the rehabilitation centers and, after qualifying, were placed in schools as craft teachers. This national policy of training and placing blind people in schools as craft instructors has continued in Ghana, and today Ghana has a relatively large number of blind persons as trained teachers in the education system. Many blind persons have moved on to become teachers in other areas.

Ghana currently has two large residential schools for the blind and two mainstream programs at the secondary level. In 1992, a mainstream program began at the elementary level as a pilot program for full integration. A teacher's training college, for the training of teachers for the blind, was developed in the 1970s by the Presbyterian church. In the 1980s the government opened its own training college for special educators. A university college for special education, including the training of teachers of the blind, was opened in 1993.

The Ghana Association of the Blind, with its new and dynamic services, has led the advocacy campaign for the rights of blind people. GAB, with member branches in all but two regions in Ghana, has a membership of several thousand blind persons. The officers are elected for a three-year term. GAB is currently led by a blind lawyer who works in the foreign service branch of the national government. GAB's National Secretariat was opened in 1995 with financial assistance from the Danish Association of the Blind.

ZAMBIA

Zambia has several blind people in important government positions and many work in salaried positions in the private sector. In 1968, a law was passed in Zambia giving protection to all people with disabilities. As frequently happens in other places, organizations of blind people were active in Zambia and their actions benefitted all disabled people. "There are five special schools in the country where 723 visually disabled children are given a primary level education" (Anonymous, 1990, p. 17). Frequently, these students attend special education programs which are attached to elementary and secondary schools. The Braille Printing House, run by the Ministry of Higher Education, prints textbooks and a special education college prepares instructors to teach. The college has four main areas of study, one of which deals with the blind and visually impaired. At one local school there are several blind teachers and a blind director.

In addition, vocational training is being offered. In 1989, 11 blind people received training allowing them to become switchboard operators. By 1990 more than 1,000 people were employed as switchboard operators in the public and private sector. At the same time, 15 blind people were employed as social workers.

There are also blind persons in high ranking government positions such as B. K. Tembo who was appointed a member of Parliament and State Minister of Culture in 1988, and R. K. Koloweka who also joined Parliament in 1988 and became governor of a district in 1990 (Anonymous, 1990, p. 18).

SOUTH AFRICA

The Republic of South Africa has the strongest economic base of African countries and the longest traditions of providing education and rehabilitation services. With the end of Apartheid, it has begun to face the challenge of making services equally available to nonwhites. Presently, much attention has been focused on bringing services to blind people living in more remote, rural regions. Dr. William Rowland, head of the South Africa National Council for the Blind (SANCB), is providing leadership and has a strong commitment to Pan-African Cooperation.

South Africa has the only residential rehabilitation center for blind people in Africa, and its services are available to clients from countries throughout Africa. South Africa, at the moment, is the only country in the region with a rehabilitation facility capable of supporting the training of regional personnel in this field. South Africa's capacity for producing Braille through its already established printing facilities meets some of the short-term needs for blind people in the region. South Africa also provides support in the production of recreational reading and fills the need for some professional literature. Furthermore, it is the only country in the region where Braille paper is produced on a commercial scale, and it has the potential for meeting nearly all of Africa's needs in this area. The South Africa National Council for the Blind (SANCB) is the only organization in the region that currently produces material which is shared with many African countries. The SANBC bimonthly magazine, *Infama*, is presently distributed throughout the continent. This magazine is the only publication that is produced within the region and is made widely available to blind adults and their organizations.

Advanced technology is also more available in South Africa. For example, the South African Society for the Blind, in collaboration with the South African National Disability Association and other private businesses, is exploring ways to make portable radios which run without batteries readily available to blind people for educational and entertainment purposes. "Turning a handle for approximately 60 seconds tightens a spring which runs a generator; one winding will power the unit for 45 minutes. These are relatively low in cost and may become extremely important to blind people in areas where literacy is low and oral traditions are strong" (Anonymous, 1996, p. 12).

ISSUES OF EMPOWERMENT IN AFRICA

Dr. William Rowland provides leadership for the South Africa National Council for the Blind. He has made a strong commitment to making rehabilitation services available in rural regions without regard to ethnic background or level of poverty. The following is an excerpt from his April 1996 presentation at the First African Forum on Rehabilitation.

Empowerment and Human Rights of Blind and Visually Impaired Persons in Africa

by Dr. William Rowland, Executive Director,
South African National Council for the Blind (SANCB)

The topic assigned to me for my keynote address is the empowerment and human rights of blind and visually impaired persons in Africa. Every term and every concept of this title could be the subject of a seminar in its own right -- empowerment–human rights–blind and visually impaired persons–in Africa; but *one* expression stands out in particular: blind and visually impaired persons. This suggests there are two categories of persons under consideration, blind people and visually impaired people. It suggests we must distinguish between the two groups, that, although they may have similar needs, they may also have differing needs and expectations. I doubt whether this distinction between blind and visually impaired persons is an African concern. The description "*visually impaired persons*" is a technical term of Western countries imposed on African culture. I shall not today examine this difference; it is perhaps an investigation for another time.

I also notice the use of the word "*persons*" rather than the word "*people*." This is altogether appropriate in a human rights context. In South Africa, we find ourselves in the middle of a constitutional debate on the question of whether protection should be given to group, language and cultural rights. The fundamental principle so far advocated in our constitutional debate is that of individual rights, the argument being that, if individual rights are protected, the other kinds of rights take care of themselves. To speak of "*blind persons*," therefore, is to focus attention on the individual. Insofar as the human rights of the blind person are protected, blind people as a group are also given protection.

Turning now to the substance of my address: What is necessary to ensure a quality life for blind persons? What factors apply and what conditions must prevail? We may also pose a second question: How do we learn the answer? How do we discover what blind people really want?

Some people will suggest we need the help of scientists or the advice of experts, field surveys and grassroots investigations. I would suggest an alternative–perhaps more effective–method. It is a method called "*listening!*" By simply listening to what people say about themselves to each other, especially in ordinary conversation, we can learn about their wishes and hopes, their problems and frustrations.

This paper very much reflects my personal impressions, but they are augmented by information gained from informal discussion groups arranged by the development workers of Ruract, a development agency of disabled persons established in the mid-1980s of which I was one of the founders. The purpose of the organisation was to promote professional services for disabled persons in rural areas; however, over time, this goal was replaced by attempts to empower disabled people and to develop grassroots organisations. When the time came when we felt this goal had been achieved, we disbanded the organisation as having completed its work. This setting, therefore, is an extra source of my material.

To return to my topic: We have to realise that the majority of blind people in Africa live in rural areas. What then are the needs expressed by blind persons living in these communities?

Let us first of all notice what needs are not expressed: mobility, equipment, and education are not mentioned. On the other hand, employment is certainly talked about because it is important to have a little money in the pocket. In other words, people do not express technical or abstract needs. The needs actually expressed arise from daily life.

Now the first and greatest need expressed is for family life. And all stages of life are intended: The child in the home, the young adult with his or her people, the married couple in relation to the older members of the family, and growing old in the family circle. One of the greatest hardships is to be separated from family; and here we must realise the impact of the removal of a blind child from the family. We know, however, that so-called special schools are seldom found in rural areas and here we learn another interesting thing. Some blind people claim that, as children, they never realised they were blind until their peers went away to school leaving them behind alone. It is hard to believe such a thing, but they speak vividly of the pain of rejection they felt at the time.

The second priority expressed by blind persons is a sexual relationship -- and what is meant is certainly a physical relationship. The belief that such matters are seldom or never discussed is false. The topic actually comes up again and again. No doubt we could analyse behavior and give all kinds of complicated explanations: Psychologists, for example, might speak of self-actualisation or self-affirmation. But, perhaps, all we are dealing with is the need to be wanted by another human being.

The third priority expressed by blind persons is employment. This is, of course, very understandable as it is the way out of poverty. In situations of high unemployment, finding a job is a haphazard business. People try to earn a little money here and a little money there, but only a permanent job or regular activity will provide reliable income. These circumstances explain why blind people with other disabled persons often get together to start self-help projects. If people can organise themselves and find some funding, they can choose a common activity or form of manufacture or assembly and generate income to be shared between the participants. Where leadership is strong and continuous, there have been some success stories. But most of these projects have failed economically. And so we need to look again at the integration of blind persons into the economic activity of the community.

Now in every community or cluster of communities there exists an opportunity network of some kind. In every community there are leaders, the community activists, and the organisers. And these are the people who give us access to the opportunities network of the community. We may engage development workers, rehabilitation workers, trainers, agricultural workers, employment finders and activists of all sorts. It is with the help of such key people that we can begin to establish the development pathway.

I would like to describe the development pathway in terms of five steps. Step one is the identification of a blind person who has the capability and wishes to enter into economic activity. Any of the agents I have mentioned may make the identification. The purpose is to refer the blind person to some resource.

The second step along the development pathway is skills training. Here I refer to the basics of so-called rehabilitation–mobility training, skills development and low-vision assistance. These are the fundamental elements of training for independence.

The third step is economic skills training. Independence skills training must come first to be followed by training in economic skills and concepts. Here people learn about buying and selling, how to provide a personal service, how to make something. The person has to learn how to set a price, how to make a profit, how to keep money records, and also about the importance of personal qualities such as reliability and trustworthiness.

Step four is choosing an economic activity. This involves the *what, where* and *how* of the personal project. The choice has to be personal but may be facilitated by the trainer, the development worker or some other competent person forming part of the process. It is at this time that we may introduce the idea of a revolving loan. To get started in some economic activity, a little money will be necessary. Therefore, a modest grant may be made, say, at the equivalent level of $100 or $200. This amount has to be repaid plus modest interest, after which the person may qualify for a further grant at a higher level. This may be repeated until the person is economically independent. Sometimes the end point may be entry into the formal economic sector.

And the final step along the development pathway—step five—is re-entry into the community to undertake an economic activity. It should be remembered we are dealing with economic activity at the grassroots level, activities such as pavement trading or house-to- house selling. From South Africa, I may mention the examples of the buying and selling of fish, the buying and selling of vegetables, of raising chickens, of shoe cleaning, of making polish, of making Vaseline, of selling stew. This is the end point of the development path which depends on the integration of blind people into a network of society, the fabric or support system of the community.

Returning to the priority of needs: The fourth need expressed by blind persons is for social relationships. Let me add a few words here about cross-disability groups. It seems that people sometimes find a special understanding for one another in a group where people have common problems. There may be more understanding for each other's situations in such a group, even more than comes from the family. There is also another consideration from a blind person's point of view—sometimes, when one is carrying out some plan or other, one gets stuck. Help from sighted persons may be needed. In a cross-disability group, people may, in fact, be more willing to help one another.

Another form of social activity that may be noted–which may seem a little unusual to mention–is singing. When blind people get together socially or travel together in a group, singing is very popular and much enjoyed. Perhaps this is why singing is also an important cultural activity. People like to organise choirs and there may be choral competitions. We also often find blind people in musical groups. This is another form of the many kinds of social relationships.

What I have been talking about are the simple elements–the basics–of ordinary life as lived and as expressed by ordinary people. These are not the priorities of scientists or social engineers but of blind people speaking from personal experience, saying what they want. It is important to try to understand and also to recognize these priorities. It seems to me, though, that we have to recognize the key element of economics. If regular income can be generated, the other things follow on naturally. Once there is income, people very quickly get married. Then the next thing is to find a place to live, preferably close to the family. It may be only a shack or a lean-to, but a place to live independently means the beginning of integration into society.

Finally then it comes to the question: What interventions are necessary to enable blind and visually impaired persons in Africa to fulfil their needs, their wishes, their expectations? To prepare people for life, we require basic services, education and rehabilitation. We may argue the merits of competing delivery systems, but the value of a quality education and training in independence skills cannot be disputed. These are fundamental provisions essential to blind people everywhere. The single most important intervention, in my opinion, is working to build the organisations of blind people, making them democratic and efficient, empowering them as our political structures and instruments of change.

Development, therefore, is not a technical process. It is a way–perhaps many ways –of making things possible. Of making it possible for people to do things for themselves. Self-development is place-finding–discovering *where* you belong, and *that* you belong. The Africa Forum is an attempt to let these things happen for blind people in Africa.

Chapter 6

BLIND PEOPLE IN THE
MIDDLE KINGDOM AND THE PEOPLE'S
REPUBLIC OF CHINA

ANCIENT CHINA

China is the most populous country in the world and can also boast its longest continuous cultural history. Blindness and the lives of blind people have changed dramatically, particularly in the country's last 150 years. This chapter reviews some of the distinctive features of the Chinese culture that influenced the development of blindness and the social arrangements permitted blind people.

There are records of notable blind people as early as the time of Confucius in the sixth century B.C.E. One of Confucius' early teachers was Ssu Song Ming, and later Confucius taught Tzu Hsia, one of his fourteen main pupils. Also, Shih K'uang was his personal musician. Finally, *Biography of Tso*, which records events during Confucian times was written by Tso Chiu, a blind scholar, during the late sixth century C.E. (Vaughan and Vaughan 1994, p. 42).

Storytelling, musical entertainment, massage, and fortune telling were occupations held by blind people even before blind guilds appeared. Historically, fortune telling has been a major vocation for blind people in China. Tradition links the origin of this work to LuT'a-I, who was a preeminent blind fortune teller and widely influential during the Han Dynasty (206 B.C.E. - 220 C.E). However, the art and craft of fortune telling and massage was not limited to China. According to Sangyeon (1994, p.5), these were viable occupations for blind people on the Korean peninsula in the same period.

Subsequently, blind massage developed as a major occupation for blind people in Japan. One reason for the large acceptance of story-telling was that it was a folk art and had appeal to both the literate and the illiterate populations. Interpreting astrological and other signs is an important elements of traditional Chinese culture, and many blind people were and are still self-employed fortune tellers.

According to Mackenzie and Flowers, "Ever since the day of Shih K'uang (the personal musician to Confucius), and probably before, the playing of musical instruments and the singing of traditional historical songs have been a particular vocation of the blind" (1947, p. 11). Musicians were paid to entertain wealthy people, or they played in public places for voluntary donations. Today, individual musicians can be seen playing in most Chinese cities, and some still occasionally play in groups. In 1991, I observed a group of more than twenty blind musicians in Gui Lin, who shared the donations from passers by. They resided in different homes in Gui Lin and had varying patterns of assistance for travel and communication as the group assembled on different days at different sights.

Guilds are organizations invented to promote the interest of members, usually but not exclusively related to crafts and occupations (Fairbank 1986; Fairbank and Feischauer 1989; French 1932; Mackenzie and Flowers 1947; Weber 1951). They have been described throughout the Middle Ages in many different parts of the world. Guilds flourished either because of local conditions or because government was unable or unwilling to protect interest groups adequately. There were guilds for merchants, bankers, carpenters, goldsmiths, blacksmiths, and those in almost every other area of economic activity.

Guilds for blind workers in China were unusual, if not unique—they involved a high degree of self-determination. Members chose their own officers and practiced self-regulation (French 1932; Mackenzie and Flowers 1947). John Burgess provides an eye witness account of a guild meeting of blind workers in Peking (Beijing) in 1919: "They were greeting their friends, discussing politics and the conditions of business, and enjoying the tea and cakes that had been provided; and it was a strange sight to see so many blind people together, each with his long bomboo cane, tapping, tapping, tapping, as they moved around the hall" (1928, p. 103). This guild held its biannual meetings to discuss politics and guild matters in a temple, unlike other guilds which had their own meeting hall. Members charged with breaking guild guidelines and rules were tried by the guild to determine guilt or innocence. Depending upon the offense, the penalty was the denial of the right to conduct business for a specified number of days. Only one of the forty-eight officers was sighted. Apprentices had to pay for their training and watch out for their own safety, while guild leaders were not responsible for accidents: "It is natural that there should be a special statement regarding accidents in the case of blind minstrels who are in danger of being run down in the streets" (Burgess 1928, p. 160).

Clearly, there was no custodialism; blind people were not cared for by professionals and their organizations were autonomous. The length of time for the apprenticeship process of guild membership usually involved three to seven years. The time varied for the different guilds according to the craft or vocation taught. As a result of their successful apprenticeship, blind people received a vocational education and permanent membership in an organization they themselves ran. In addition, occupational guilds were organized and operated in a manner similar to that of other guilds in Chinese society. Whatever else sighted people thought of the blind, they at least observed them working in occupations that were both legitimate and venerable and which were organized in the same manner that work was organized for the sighted.

The apprentice system paved the way for privately run schools in which thousands of blind people were trained as fortune tellers. In addition, schools developed to train musicians and beggars. The competence of blind persons to provide services, as well as their traditional claims to particular occupations, was widely recognized. During the 1930s, fortune tellers could earn as much as one thousand dollars per month in Shanghai currency (Fryer 1942, p. 155).

THE MODERN ERA

China experienced tremendous levels of social change during the social, political, and economic revolution culminating during the period 1949-1976. The government, directed by the Chinese Communist Party, began to instill new secular, socialist values and to promote social arrangements for China in an attempt to change almost everything associated with its feudal past. Under a system of strict state control, new forms of education, employment, and social organization developed. As far as it could be accomplished by the state, there was an intentional break with the past. Change was made by revolutionary decree. As a means of control, all social organizations now involved state sponsorship. In each organization a member of the Chinese Communist Party, a cadre or party secretary, was appointed to represent the interest of the party. As a result, autonomous organizations of blind workers, as well as all other autonomous organizations, ceased to exist.

Under Chairman Mao, campaigns were launched to rid China of its feudal, dynastic past. For example, at the beginning of the Cultural Revolution in 1966, the Anti Four Olds Campaign urged young revolutionaries to destroy old thought, old culture, old customs, and old habits (Salisbury 1992). The Cultural Revolution (1966 to 1976) was a nationwide intense attack on what Mao judged to be lingering influences of the old order. During that period, fortune telling, one of the most traditional occupations for the blind, had a difficult time. Any activity considered superstitious and associated with the feudal past was criticized and its proponents punished. Individuals could be beaten and publicly humiliated in "struggle" or "self criticism" sessions. Blind fortune tellers were not exempt: "These specialists (often blind people covertly supplementing their meager income by this activity) are not criticized most of the time, but some have been dragged out for struggle meetings during intensive campaigns, and put out of business temporarily or permanently" (Parish & Whyte 1978, p. 254). The rise of modern socialist China affected many blind people in two major ways—autonomous organizations were no longer permitted and the occupations themselves, except blind massage, were discredited. Begging was not appropriate in a society with an egalitarian, socialist ideology.

In the totalitarian state of modern Socialist China with its totalitarian state, life was difficult for its blind citizens. There were no special institutions, professional interest groups, or organizations competing for the blindness domain. With the political, economic, and social revolution, change was imposed on blind people and their organizations arbitrarily, from the top down. There were no interest groups providing specialized services for blind people. The only exceptions were schools founded by Western Christian missionaries around 1850.

However, the schools educated relatively few blind people. The tradition still exists in Taiwan.

Since 1982 under the leadership of Deng Xiaoping, China has entered a period of economic reform which includes movement towards a free market economy and borrowing ideas and technology from other countries. How have blind people fared during this recent period of Chinese history?

One occupational area that has both flourished and attracted government support is blind massage. In 1988, the People's Republic of China issued the first Five Year Plan for the rehabilitation of handicapped people. Although it had relatively little to say about blindness, the plan considered blind massage an occupation worthy of governmental support. As a result, China has now increased the number of professional schools, and blind massage is a significant occupational field for blind people (Zhang 1990, p. 2). In a 1992 official government report, the authors state that there are more than 800 massage hospitals and clinics employing approximately 8,000 blind massage therapists (Progress Report on 8th Five Year Plan). Each has professional status and his or her title is "doctor." From the perspective of Western tradition, we might say that they reside in sheltered workshops; yet, the conditions they endure and the pay and respect they receive are better, in most cases, than what blind people in the United States experience in most sheltered workshops.

There are other signs that the quality of life for blind people in China is improving. Now there are national days to recognize competitions among disabled athletes, much like those for the Special Olympics in the United States. Also, the government advocates the removal of architectural barriers "whenever feasible" (Chen 1992). China participates in and hosts international conferences about disability.

Whether in the United States or any other country, such efforts and programs are good for business. Whatever China does for the blind and physically disabled, such programs attract funding, consultants, and teachers from outside China, and they offer economic opportunities for those providing them. Economics and politics are the most useful vantage points for understanding these developments because they integrate the changing situation of blind people with changes in the structure of Chinese economy and society.

It is difficult to determine the employment level of blind people in China. Clearly, some have relatively high paying jobs, such as the 8,000 working in blind massage; however, a 1988 nationwide government survey indicated that there were 7,550,000 blind people in China. Unemployment data are not available. If only one-half of China's reported blind population is of working age, a relatively small percentage work in blind massage and other government-sponsored jobs. As in most societies, work opportunities are least available in rural and small town areas. In the government-directed sector of the economy, incentives make it easier in China than in the United States to create jobs for handicapped people (Gang 1991). For example, government policy now eliminates or reduces taxes on businesses owned by disabled people or by those employing significant numbers of disabled workers. The cultural and social differences between rural and urban China are great, and government-created employment and educational opportunities are more readily available in urban areas (Chen, 1992).

From 1949 until 1982, the planned Chinese economy emphasized infrastructure development. Government-sponsored programs for those with disabilities were a low priority. Specialized programs, specialized schools, specialized concerns, and Western-based cultural ideas about the individual primarily had come to China in small doses because of Western missionary activities throughout the hundred years preceding 1949. Such efforts were not only different from traditional customs, they were also associated with the era of economic and political exploitation by the West. However, a humanistic tradition is now developing in China in a manner which illustrates how important one person's contribution can be.

In his article, "Changing Beliefs About Disability in Developing Countries," Mallory observes: "In general, variations in social attitudes are thought to be associated with economic conditions, the state of medical and therapeutic technology, social policies (and their relation to conceptions of human rights), religious and cultural belief systems, and idiosyncratic factors such as the role of political leaders who take a personal interest in the lives of people with disabilities" (1993, p. 1). China well illustrates the last condition. There has been no more powerful person than Deng Xiao Ping in China during the past 20 years. His son, Deng Pu Fang, who was educated as a physicist, was injured in a fall and paralyzed from the waist down amid the activity of a hostile crowd during the Cultural Revolution. "Pu Fang's long struggle with his crippled body had turned his mind to the human condition in a philosophical way not often found among Chinese. He had become a passionate believer in humanitarianism and resolved to devote his life to helping his fellow men" (Salisbury 1992, p. 419). In the initial absence of government support, Deng Pufang began to raise money through private appeals and established the China Welfare Fund for the Handicapped. His important father gave him entry to "high places." His efforts brought about the rapid development of the China Disabled Persons' Association and factories created to employ handicapped people.

However, humanistic concerns are not yet widespread in China. Economic interests are the dominant factor in explaining China's rapid development of programs for disabled people. I was told that entrepreneurs employ disabled people to take advantage of government incentives. Skeptics criticized Deng Rifany for creating a large number of factories and related businesses which, while providing some employment opportunity for people with disabilities, are providing even more economic opportunities for the able-bodied who frequently manage them. This situation is little different from that available to the people well employed as directors of agencies or managers of sheltered workshops in Western societies. To encourage equality for the disabled, the United Nations designated the years of 1983 to 1992 as the Decade of Disabled Persons. Even though cooperation frequently leads to economic assistance by countries outside China, the People's Republic has started many programs which, to a marked degree, parallel those in more economically advanced societies.

THE REHABILITATION BUSINESS IN CHINA

Economically-based interest groups are a feature of China's developing free market economy. A United States based foundation sponsored by former President Carter recently provided funds for a new factory in Beijing, which produces prosthetic devices. Associated with China's Disabled Person's Association, many factories have been created to afford employment opportunities for disabled people. Monies to improve existing institutions are also obtained from the World Bank, the United Nations, and other private agencies. For example, in

1992, a United Nations program funded a modern educational building at The School for Deaf and Blind Children in Xi'an. Within the
large and rapidly growing Chinese economy, enterprises and programs related to disability are relatively insignificant. However, as in
the West, they are important to the privileged individuals who control
these economic resources.

In China, unlike the United States, all programs for the disabled,
except the few supported by philanthropic organizations from outside
China, are under the lone government sponsored umbrella organization, The China Disabled People's Federation, which is controlled by
one person. China has not developed a distinct subprofession to serve
its blind citizens. However, during the past sixteen years of economic
reform and openness to the West, China has established institutions
and programs which loosely parallel most of those in the United States
and other Western countries. Except for the limited missionary influence mentioned above, they did not exist prior to 1949. However,
they have flourished under China's economic free market modemiza-
tion and are best understood in the context of China's recent capitalist developments.

Not only is China developing similar programs, the consequences
for blind people are also similar. To illustrate, I will comment briefly
on my interviews with "ordinary" blind people living under these new
conditions.

OBSERVING BLINDNESS IN CHINA

During the past four years, I have made three trips to the People's
Republic of China, ranging in length from six weeks to nine months,
which included teaching at the Xi'an Foreign Language University in
Shaanxi Province. With the exception of Northeast China, I have visited almost every province and autonomous region.

I took every opportunity to learn about the conditions of blind people and rehabilitation practices in the People's Republic of China. I
interviewed social workers, school administrators and teachers, government officials, and fifty-two "ordinary" blind people (by "ordinary,"
I mean not employed by the state). Of the fifty-two, only three were
women. Therefore, the interviews do not represent a random sample.

With only one exception, I did not seek governmental permission. I used the goodwill of friends, acquaintances,and interpreters to arrange informal interviews. For example, when arriving in a new city, I would first go to the government-sponsored tourist office and make arrangements to employ an interpreter/tour guide. I would then explain my interest in talking with blind people and my desire to visit schools, blind massage clinics and so on. As far as I could tell, I was never denied access to any location. With the exception of those in blind massage clinics, I met the fifty-two blind people through random encounters on the street, which presented an interesting problem. Large crowds gathered to figure out why a foreigner would want to talk to a blind person. I quickly developed a new strategy. When we encountered a blind person, I would go to a nearby restaurant or park bench and my interpreter would return and explain to blind musicians or fortune tellers that a foreigner would like to talk to them about their experiences with blindness in China and would be happy to compensate for lost revenue if they would do so in a quieter location. Some individuals declined, apparently not believing the offer or not willing to vacate their place. It would have been impossible in terms of time, resources, government permission, and the absence of specific lists to have obtained any type of random sample. I visited several schools for blind and deaf children and several clinics where people are employed in blind massage. In addition to reading the small amount of relevant material available in English, I used translators to review several journals and government documents.

Understanding or interpreting blindness in one's own society is difficult enough; it is infinitely more so in a totally different culture, particularly when interpreters are necessary. To illustrate, during my first visit to one of Xi'an's two schools for blind and deaf children, I asked the principal why there were no blind teachers. He answered that such teachers did not know enough. However, he kindly observed that his school would be happy to employ someone like me. Although I had a good interpreter, I did not learn until the next visit that we had both misunderstood: the principal meant that blind people could not know enough because an appropriate education was not available to them.

On another occasion I informally visited the residence of several blind people whose unit worked at a blind massage clinic. They described different ways they had experienced discrimination, including being laughed at or taunted when they stumbled while walking down the street, and having no opportunities to advance in their occupation. Two days later, I met the sighted officials of this clinic in a formally arranged meeting. Subsequently, the director took me on a tour which included a clinic where several blind massage therapists were at work. While I was receiving a complimentary massage, the director invited me to ask questions of the workers. Unbeknown to the director, one of these therapists was the man who had described various kinds of discrimination to me two days earlier. To the same question and in a very straight-faced manner, he told me, in the presence of the director and party secretary for the work unit, "There has been no discrimination in China against blind people since 1949." I cannot claim that the fifty-two individuals I interviewed comprised a random sample; however, I was struck by the consistency of their responses. I always asked: "How do you benefit or how are you helped by programs sponsored by China's Disabled People's Federation?" Almost everyone said, "Not at all." They observed that those who benefitted were "well connected"; that is, they were from prominent or wealthy families or had been in the army. I am not trying to minimize the importance of the employment opportunities that have been created; however, the economic interests of these programs result in stratification patterns among blind people, which have also been described in the United States (Scott 1969). Agencies appreciate clients who are appealing and likely to be successful: it helps with fund raising. People who cooperate and present themselves well have more opportunities to participate in visible, higher status organizational positions than less favored blind people.

A few individuals even commented that they had been much better off before the recent free market reforms. In a work brigade or commune, they had been given tasks "to do" and lived as well as others in their units. Now, if they are not among the privileged blind, they are on their own. I discussed employment with several men who were doing blind massage of the upper body, using stools and working on the street near tourist hotels. Two such men in Kuming told me that they preferred working on the street to working at a blind hospital because they could earn more money and were not "bossed around." I asked if there was anything negative about working alone. They replied that sometimes they were forced to leave their sites when a public meeting or occasion might cause local officials to clear the street of beggars or disabled people doing any kind of work.

Certainly, our cultural values concerning people with disabilities are different from those of both Imperial and modern China. Yet, with the development of the free market economy in China, striking similarities have appeared between rehabilitation programs in both cultures. These similarities revolve around the economic organizations, the resources they represent, and the career opportunities for those administrators and employees who run programs for the blind and other handicapped people. To date, blind and disabled people in China have not raised the issue of "empowerment;" this will doubtless be a late stage in China's future political development. The following charts summarize the major distinctions between the social and cultural arrangements for blind people in China and the West through history.

Table 3. Prior to 1911.

China (Imperial Feudal Era)	*United States*
• No special schools or asylums	• Specialized institutions for the blind
• Autonomous guilds for blind workers	• Humanitarian concerns for separate blind people for specialized education • Custodial treatment • No independent organizations of blind people
• No humanistic tradition (no "nobless oblige")	• Proliferation of private philanthropic agencies to provide services to blind people

Table 4. 1911-1978.

China	*United States*
• Social, political and economic revolution • Emergence of totalitarian	• Science used to provide "objective" information to explain the specialized problems of blindness • Workers for the blind in the process of establishing a profession (The Progressive Ear)
• Disappearance of automous guilds of blind people	• First nationwide automous organization of blind people • National Federation of the Blind established in 1940
• Disappearance of civil society • All organizations under CCP supervision	• Proliferation of private philanthropic organizations • Groups contend in civil society for funding, legitimation and different approaches to rehabilitation and education
Education and other programs for blind people developed with tight political control	• Claims-making activity concerning mainstreaming and "full inclusion"
• Five Year Plans approved at highest level	• Autonomous organizations of blind people promote self advocacy and equal treatment
• No independent consumer groups	• Conflict between professional and consumer groups over rehabilitation goals and policies

Table 5. 1978-Present.

China	United States
• Borrowing of technology and program ideas from the West	• MA and Ph.D. degrees available in blindness rehabilitation • Business proliferated to create electronic and other appliances for blind people
• One umbrella organization created for all disability groups	• Licensing of professionals who work for the blind • Occupational specialization throughout public and private agencies
• The China Disabled People's Organization controlled by one man, son of nation's most powerful person	• Intense efforts by organizations of blind people for self-determination • Conflict with organized professionals
• Early stages of independent programs funded from outside China	• Independent organizations of blind people create and run their own rehabilitation programs • Many private agencies develop international programs
• China moving toward free-market economy and civil society	• More then 800 agencies and programs compete for government and philanthropic economic resources • Rehabilitation is big business
• Programs for disabled represent new economic resources and opportunities	• Continued growth in public and private funding for rehabilitation programs • Americans With Disabilities Act

THE FIRST FIVE-YEAR PLAN CONCERNING PEOPLE WITH DISABILITIES

In response to the initiatives sponsored by the United Nations' concern for improving the lives of people with disabilities and partly from the leadership of Deng Pu Fang, son of Deng Xiao Ping, China has made public policy commitments intended to benefit them, including blind people. The first Five-Year Plan for centrally-directed economic development began in 1958. Adapted from the experience of the USSR, it is regularly used for planning in many areas of Chinese society. In 1988, the People's Republic of China (PRC) published its first Five-Year Plan for the rehabilitation and education of people with disabilities.

Table 6 compiles information from a national survey of the prevalence of various types of disabilities in China (Vaughan, 1993 b). The data base resulted from a sample survey that

Table 6. Educational Attainment by Disability Category.

Category	Blind	Deaf	Disabled	Multiple Disabilities
College				
Number	15,100	56,600	36,200	18,100
%	0.2	0.32	0.48	0.27
Senior				
Number	71,000	267,300	358,600	36,300
%	0.94	1.51	4.75	0.54
Junior				
Number	297,500	1,054,900	1,198,200	177,000
%	3.94	5.96	15.87	2.63
Primary				
Number	1,211,800	3,991,400	2,338,200	819,000
%	16.05	22.55	30.93	12.17
Illiterate				
Number	5,954,700	12,328,100	3,621,700	6,738,400
%	78.87	69.65	47.79	84.39

included 369,816 households containing 1,579,314 individuals. Nearly one in five of these households contained at least one person with a disability and 4.9 percent of all individuals had some type of disabling condition. The results projected a population of approximately 51,640,000 persons with disabilities (Work Plan 1988). Table 6 indicates the total number of individuals in each disability category as revealed by the sample survey. The table also contains the level of education attainment by disability grouping (Education, 1989).

New talk planning processes occurred at all levels: counties, cities, and provinces held meetings to determine the content of the first Five-Year Plan, not unlike the many conferences that preceded the White House Conferences on Aging in the United States. The initiative came from the highest level of government in Beijing, which requested that each province and autonomous region obtain ideas from local governments concerning the needs of people with disabilities. The result was the drafting of a final document which provincial leaders presented to the State council; the result was the first Five-Year Plan. I learned about this process from interviews with provincial government officials, some of whom participated directly in it. I met with them without specific government approval in advance, and at that time, 1991-92, informants did not wish to be identified.

The Five-Year Plan concentrates on encouraging government to improve educational opportunities and special programs for disabled people. It emphasizes mainstreaming whenever possible and expanding programs for special education teachers. The plan includes the development of new technology for the enhanced functioning of people with disabilities and making appropriate medical intervention a high priority.

Most of the policies are stated in general terms, particularly those related to blindness. Specific goals are nearly absent, with the exception of the proposal to perform 500,000 cataract operations before the end of the term. An unspecified increase of the number of clinics providing blind massage is also a goal. The Five-Year Plan specifically states that the economic resources for "improving the cause of people with disabilities" will be available only in direct relationship to growth in the national economy. Funds will not be diverted from other government activities (Work Plan, 1988).

In general, the Plan appeals to all levels of government for improvements in employment, health and education, and the welfare of disabled individuals. The document states that disabled people are to be treated justly and fairly, in accordance with the tenets of socialist humanism. Also, it describes the responsibility of society to look out for the interests of people with disabilities. In turn, disabled people are urged to observe the laws and practices of society and live up to its moral standards. The Plan's message to people with disabilities is one of optimism, self-confidence, and self-respect. Further, it expects them to be as independent as possible and to contribute to the construction of a socialist society.

NEW LAWS TO PROTECT PEOPLE WITH DISABILITIES

In 1990, the national government of the People's Republic of China issued a new official document in a language and style almost identical to the Five-Year Plan discussed above. The new legislation, entitled "Law of the People's Republic of China in the Protection of Disabled Persons," was not specifically mandated by the Plan, but it is consistent with the general intent. This legislation developed through the advocacy efforts of the Disabled People's Federation and sympathetic provincial and national officials.

The document instructs schools to admit qualified students with disabilities and tells employers to give them work opportunities. The document also encourages society to provide access to all areas of cultural life, for example, by making Braille available for blind persons. In addition, public services within society should give priority to people with disabilities for the use of these services, including transportation. People who are blind should not be charged when using buses, trollies, subways or ships (Laws 1990, p. 16). Nor should there be a charge for mailing reading material to people who are blind. Thus, China now reciprocates with the international community in the free mailing of materials for blind people. In specific laws promulgated by this new document, people who are blind are exempted from obligatory work, especially pursuits required to help specific state projects, and from mandatory fees to support welfare services. If a person with a disability is maltreated by one who is in any way responsible for his or her care, the caregiver would be subject to prosecution under Act 22 of the new legal code for the People's Republic of China (Laws, 1990, p. 19).

Law 145 provides a prison term of three years for those who publicly insult persons with disabilities; however, this is only enforced if the insulted person appeals to the court for justice. This process of appeal is costly and complicated and not likely to result in litigation.

The legal profession and the justice system were nearly eliminated during the decade of the Cultural Revolution (1966-1976). Now lawyers are in demand to serve China's rapidly developing free market economy. However, it would be very difficult for an ordinary blind person to use the new laws to seek justice or equal opportunity. Most people with disabilities are poor and have few connections with those in powerful positions. Without them, the probability of receiving justice is minimal.

The first Five-Year Plan and the new laws described above seldom apply explicitly to blind people. Exceptions are the goal of 500,000 cataract operations and expanded employment opportunities in blind massage. The education students receive in schools for the blind is not comparable to that received by students in the public schools. Therefore, despite a change in the laws, it is almost impossible for blind students to be competitive in the national examinations which lead to public higher education. Private schools are now developing at both secondary and higher levels (Vaughan 1996). This situation may provide additional opportunities for some blind students whose families can afford the cost of private education.

There appears to be more employment opportunities for the deaf and mobility handicapped. In principle, placing people with disabilities in occupations is easier in China than in the United States. The government can encourage placement by direct and significant economic incentives to factories and other work units employing people with disabilities, and many do so. However, except for those in blind massage, there are relatively few employment opportunities for the visually impaired.

In general, socialist humanism attempts to "take care of" Chinese citizens. For example, since 1949 the People's Republic of China has greatly reduced prostitution and begging, and government programs have expanded employment opportunities for people with disabilities. The first Five-Year Plan and the new protection laws provided a framework for directing future government efforts. It also encouraged the borrowing of technology and new ideas about rehabilitation and special education. China currently has more than thirty programs which are sponsored by organizations outside the country. Most of these are described by Mindes (1991, pp. 8-39).

National programs may be further improved by the recent political integration of Hong Kong into the People's Republic of China. The Hong Kong Society for the Blind has received technical and economic support from Western organizations for years. The Hong Kong Society has grown and become one of the leaders in Asian regional cooperation. "In its 40 years of service, the HKSB has always maintained very good relationships with overseas organizations in the West, serving the visually impaired, such as the Christoffel Blindness Mission, Perkins School for the Blind, the Royal Institute for the Blind, etc." (Chan 1996, p. 19). The author goes on to cite three reasons for its successes: the availability of Western information and technology, well-trained staff, and strong ties to overseas organizations serving the visually impaired. In the past decade the Hong Kong Society has cooperated with the China Disabled Persons Federation (CDPF) in many ways. It has provided links between China and overseas technical and economic resources, staff training, and development opportunities including recent technological developments, and new ideas and project proposals for joint cooperation. These have included progress in the prevention of blindness, vocational training, staff training, education of the visually impaired, modernization of Braille production equipment, and so on.

Cooperation has benefitted both. The Hong Kong Society has learned from the Disabled People's Federation about training and opportunity employment in blind massage. In fact, China hosted an international conference on blind massage in Xi'an in 1992 and a research-oriented conference in Gou Muchi in 1996. From its outset, the Federation has been generic. All programs are administered under the one organization directed by Deng Pu Fang. Each district, province and major city has an agency subordinate to the national organization. Unfortunately, programs dealing with blindness are combined with all others. Except for those in schools, there are few specialized programs for the blind and visually impaired. While in China at different times (1991-1994), I concluded that blindness was in a weak position relative to other areas of disability. Chan reports that this situation is changing. Services to the visually impaired have greatly improved, and in 1990,the Federation established a Department of the Blind. Programs for blind people have had much greater viability with the leadership of Mr. Xu Bailum. He developed the Gold Key Program, which provides teacher training and other support to promote Chinese Braille literacy.

Gender is an important element in any culture, and no less so for blind men and women. Patterns of gender segregation, discrimination, and exploitation also vary to the extent societies have become industrially modernized. Modernization does not eliminate gender differences; they simply take new forms. To illustrate, I conclude this chapter with the following article, included here with the permission of *The Educator*. In it, Cordelia Scharpf, a blind woman from the United States, describes her recent experience with blind girls and women in various settings in the People's Republic of China.

Education of the Blind in the People's Republic of China: Attending Classes in Seven Schools for the Blind and Meeting Blind Chinese Women (1996)

Visiting the People's Republic of China for the first time last May and June, I sought first to learn about the situation of blind Chinese girls and women, particularly their educational and vocational opportunities, and second, being partially of Chinese (Taiwanese) decent myself, I wanted to learn more about my Chinese heritage. With the kind help of my friend, L. Campbell of Overbrook School for the Blind of Philadelphia, PA, Mr. W. Brohier from Malaysia, president of the International Council of Educators of the Visually Impaired, Mrs. G. Chan, president of the Hong Kong Society for the Blind, and members of Amity Foundation of Nanjing, PRC, I was able to contact principals of seven schools for the blind in China. I was allowed to visit their schools and interview select groups of girl students. I was also fortunate to meet blind women working at a massage hospital in Beijing, the Braille Press near Beijing, and at the home of a blind Japanese woman teaching Japanese to blind young adults in Tienjing.

Accompanied by my interpreter-cum-guide, I traveled by train or plane on Saturdays and explored cities on foot on Sundays—once walking a distance of about 13 miles of the east-west-axis in Shanghai, and another time walking the north-south-axis of the second city ring of Beijing. I could witness a lot through hearing, smelling and touching, and my guide's very vivid descriptions of our surroundings and activities served to enliven my perceptions of things Chinese." I quickly learned not to venture out by myself. There were not only vehicles of all kinds, whose drivers used horns rather than brakes, but also the notorious throngs of people milling through busy streets. First my guide and I waited patiently for the traffic to slow down to cross streets, but then decided to "do as the Romans do": we pushed along with the crowd and trusted that bike riders and drivers saw us in time. Even with a guide it was strenuous for me to navigate on China's streets filled with loud traffic noise and aromas from countless food stalls. The acoustic and olfactory markers with which I usually orient myself were now my worst enemies.

From Mondays through Fridays, from about 8 A.M. to 3 P.M., we sat in classes observing students and teachers engage in their lessons. Every school day began with morning ceremonies in which principals reminded students of particular charges for the day, emphasizing patriotism and devotion to the Party. Between classes students did gymnastics, accompanied by loud music, to loosen up. These exercises took place in courtyards, or on rainy days, in hallways. On average, students did gymnastics three to five times a day, in addition to classes in physical education. The school for the blind in Shanghai still prides itself for assigning rope jumping as a comprehensive exercise to strengthen muscles and lung capacity, and improve coordination.

I observed classes in grade and middle schools, as well as vocational schools (mostly massage therapy, but also piano tuning). In Qingdao, I visited the one and only high school for the blind in China. The students in the schools I visited were very well-behaved and diligent.

Memorizing facts, lyrics and formulae in natural sciences characterized the style of learning. Teaching natural sciences was both inductive and deductive: after working on examples, teachers dictated principles and formulae which students memorized and were expected to use through their school lives. Patiently, students wrote lengthy and complicated formulae with styluses and slates. In most cases, English instruction (the only foreign language taught) was based on grammar translation, rather than more modern and diversified teaching methods. The schools made use of language laboratories, trying to improve the students' pronunciation. Some students listened to BBC or Voice of America at 6 A.M. to improve their English. What delighted me was the fact that they studied the international Music Braille at an early age and could read music scores and have a sizable repertoire of songs and instrumental music.

Students learn to use the slates and styluses in first grade or whenever they transfer from regular schools to schools for the blind. I was very impressed by the speed of their writing Braille onto magazines they "recycled" as notebooks. They ably and correctly "drew" shapes in plane geometry by using their slates and rulers. In Beijing, parents and teachers designed compasses. The school often had only a small number of charts and diagrams, which were not part of students' textbooks. The textbooks are Braille versions of those used by their sighted peers and are produced by the Braille press in Shanghai.

During breaks or afternoon sessions, teachers shared with me their pedagogical and methodological insights and inquired about the educational and vocational situation of the blind in Germany and the United States. They were especially interested in mobility training, technological advances for the blind, and mainstreaming of blind children. Since the early 1990s under the auspices and pedagogical supervision of the *Golden Key Project*, an increasing number of blind children has been mainstreamed in primary schools in their communities. The *Golden Key Project* trains local teachers to teach blind students, introduces them to Chinese Braille, and gives material support.

Select groups of students from middle and vocational schools patiently answered my questions about their lives, their vocational opportunities and hopes for their future. We spent many very insightful hours reflecting on the similar tasks we have to master, such as mobility, cooking, sewing and more. I especially enjoyed meeting the high school students in Qingdao. They wish to enroll at university but are denied entrance on the basis of their visual impairment. All students must pass entrance examinations in order to enroll at high schools or universities in China. The examination also includes a test of the applicant's visual acuity. In the case of severely visually impaired and blind students, their visual impairment prevents them from being considered as candidates. However, since 1987, the special division for handicapped students at the University in Changchun, Northeastern Province, has offered blind students courses in massage therapy, music, Chinese literature and Chinese medicine to train them as teachers in schools for the blind, practioners or performers. The principal of the school for the blind in Qingdao is currently negotiating with the Commission of Education on local and national levels to open other universities to visually impaired students.

Those students who do not pass the entrance examination to vocational schools or the special division at the University of Changchun work at "sheltered factories" doing assembly work. Some can work at the Braille Press in Shanghai and Beijing as proofreaders. There are no official statistics for the unemployment rate among blind people in China. Principals of schools for the blind must try harder to place graduating students. Especially after the Opening, massage therapy is no longer reserved for blind people exclusively. Competition for jobs is keen and connections are needed to find employment.

Meeting blind girl students and women at work gave me an invaluable opportunity to learn about their educational and vocational possibilities. Women students generally represent about one-third of the student body at the schools I visited. They did the same tasks as boys and performed well, academically speaking, including in natural sciences. They are expected to internalize: all procedures needed in home management, crafts and sports. I was impressed by their stamina and endurance in sprinting, swimming and other highly competitive disciplines. When I met them, they were preparing in extracurricular courses for the Paralympics this summer in Atlanta and for national competitions among the schools for the blind.

They shared with me their awareness and frustration of being the first ones to lose jobs in times of recession, downsizing and tough competition. They know from older sisters and friends about prostitution at the workplace of massage therapists in southern China, about many who are unemployed and become burdens for their families, and about feeling isolated once they leave school and must solve problems on their own. One of the women I met spoke of her difficulties finding a job after she lost her eyesight while working as an English teacher. Although she had mastered Braille and could continue to teach, no school offered her a position despite openings. Like some other blind women and men, she is learning Japanese in the hope of enrolling at a Japanese university to further her education and improve chances for employment in China. Having talked with young blind Chinese people and partly shared their daily routine, I now understand the circumstances they are confronted with. I hope that their educational and vocational opportunities will improve, that they will have the same opportunities as their sighted peers and mainstream themselves more fully in their society.

Chapter 7

SPAIN'S UNIQUE ORGANIZATION–THE ORGANIZACIÓN NACIONAL DE CIEGOS ESPAÑOLES (ONCE)

Humans create objects, ideas and organizations. Many creations never become important, while others are modified, built upon and sometimes incorporated as prominent features of a society. Blind people, with the help of a few others, have established such an organization in Spain. Throughout the world, there is none comparable to the Spanish National Organization of the Blind–the Organización Nacional de Ciegos Españoles (ONCE), and blindness in modern Spain cannot be understood without learning about the ONCE.

HISTORICAL BACKGROUND

Like those in France and China during the Middle Ages, Spanish blind people organized themselves into guilds for mutual benefit and self-protection. For example, a brotherhood of blind men was founded in Barcelona in 1339. The Spanish guilds, like those in China, controlled certain functions such as the saying of house prayers (Garvía, 1996).

In a similar manner, the blind in Madrid enjoyed two monopolies: the sale of the Gaceta and other official leaflets and newspapers (such as *El correo de Madrid*, called for this reason, *"El correo de los Ciegos,"*("The Blindmen's Post"), and the musical performances in the streets of the city (at which the blind sold their own literature, popularly called *pliegos de cordel* or *pliegos de ciegos*. (p. 493)

167

However, the Age of Enlightenment and the spread of the idea of a free market economy led to the demise of guilds in Spain. The outcry against monopolies associated with the dominance of a free market capitalist economy affected all guilds, including those of blind people. In addition, public campaigns against begging contributed to their decline (p. 493).

With the disruption of the guild system, the nineteenth century saw Spain follow the pattern of most European countries and the United States of America. Special schools to teach vocations and "poorhouses" were created. In 1857, a law provided for local schools for blind students. However, Spain was weak economically and there was very little money for these schools or residences. It was not until the 1860s that Spain's leading school, in Madrid, had more than twenty people. In fact, by the turn of the century, there were only one hundred thirty-six blind high school graduates in all of Spain.

Professor Garvía (1996), summarizes two major social conditions which contributed to the successful transformation of the social situation of blind people in Spain.

> There are two reasons which can explain this "great transformation" of the Spanish blind. Firstly, the fiscal crisis of local governments during the 19th Century and the financial difficulties of the Church (which was forced to sell a significant portion of its real estate), did not allow for the creation of poorhouses, or workhouses for the blind (or in general for the poor, see Castro 1990, and Tedde 1994). Neither was there in Spain a strong middle class with a tradition of charity to substitute for the state and the Church. Thus, the Spanish blind were left wandering and begging in the cities, giving them a chance to retain their own formal and informal associations.
>
> Secondly, Spanish neutrality during the Great War allowed the Spanish state to escape from the need to set up welfare and employment programs for the blind, which the belligerent countries needed to meet the demands of their blind veterans (and eventually, those of the civilian blind). The Spanish blind were given a new chance to strengthen their own organisations and to make of the Spanish peninsula an impressive laboratory in which local organisations were forced to experiment with different occupational solutions to the problem of begging (such as the sale of water in Andalusia, the musical performances in the streets, or the sale of popular literature—*pliegos de ciegos*). (p. 505)

The secondary schools that trained the few blind graduates were creating a source of future leadership. During this period the Spanish economy was in disarray and poverty became concentrated in urban areas as rural people moved to the city seeking opportunity. Many people besides the blind were begging. Educated blind people provided leadership for informal organizations of blind people that persisted after the demise of the former guilds (Garvía, 1996, pp. 493-494).

> That there were informal organisations of the blind is not surprising, since mendicancy in large cities had never been an individual practice, but rather a practice (or occupation) loosely organised and structured through hierarchies, specialisations and demarcations of territory which, consequently, gave an advantage to the organised. (p. 494)

The first legally recognized organization for blind people after the period of the guilds was formed in 1882 in Madrid. Former graduates of the Madrid School for the Blind, in 1894, created another organization, *Centro Protectivo e Instructor de Ciegos.* The educated leadership of this organization criticized the special schools for the blind and the policy that resulted in forced segregation. According to a Spanish source in 1908, leadership viewed blind people thus:

> After so many centuries of charity . . . the blind today do not have any other recourse than begging. [The blind] are educated in organized special schools in order that later they are secluded in squalid sewers that the charitable spirit call asylums, but which cannot accommodate not only the average poor, but not even the last being disposed with a shred of dignity and the slightest spark of reason. (Asamblea, 1908, p. 337)

The political response to this criticism was the creation of a national public trust whose responsibility was care for the deaf and "abnormal." Beginning in 1910, the trust underwent six reorganizations by 1930, and the results were disappointing to most blind people in Spain. These trusts had little power and were dominated by bureaucrats, physicians, and educators. During this period, a survey revealed the sorry state of blind people and programs intended for their benefit. According to a 1913 report, "Organisations of the blind, which existed in most cities visited, were dedicated almost exclusively to begging. Most of the special schools lacked resources or had already been closed" (Garvía, 1996, p. 495). Subsequently, the National Federation of the Blind was founded in 1924, and it asked the government for a new national trust which would be adequately funded and which would include blind people in the decision-making process.

Most blind people in Spain were frustrated by the welfare policies of Primo de Rivera's dictatorship (1923-1930), which intended to isolate blind people from the rest of society. For example, Martinez Anido wanted to use the government monies to create three large asylums, "residences," as the means of dealing with beggars (Garvía, 1994, pp. 20-21). Under dictatorial conditions, blind people cautiously opposed this approach, which led to the creation of Federación Hispánica de Ciegos (Spanish Federation of the Blind) in 1932. Under the Second Republic (1931-1936), blind people were included in the decision-making process. "The 1934 Trust began its activities in a way that satisfied the blind: it conducted a census of the blind, created three vocational workshops, subsidised three orchestras, provided pensions for one hundred elderly in Madrid, and subsidised, in a small way, two organisations of the blind" (p. 496). However, because the overall performance of the trust was poor, blind people concluded that, rather than counting on the state, they should solve their own problems.

The 1930s saw much ferment in developing organizations for the blind in both the United States and Europe. Blinded war veterans had aspirations other than begging. Some leaders thought that mechanized forms of assembly line production might offer new employment opportunities (Garvía, 1994).

> In the thirties there were many Italian, French, German, English and North American blind veterans who were working at full capacity and in the same conditions as the sighted workers in Fiat, Siemens, Renault, Ford and other large companies; and in the same years many blind Spaniards placed their hopes in the mechanization of industry. (p. 24)

On the other hand, the large numbers of loosely organized blind beggars wanted to preserve their livelihoods. Some of these groups created illegal lotteries in eastern Spain during this period (Garvía, 1996, p. 496), but they were poorly organized and fraud was frequently alleged. A successful lottery was established by blind people in Barcelona in 1934. In fact, the philosophy and success of the ONCE was foreshadowed in the success of the Barcelona lottery. "With the proceeds from this lottery, the blind of Barcelona created their own vocational training workshop, a special school and a Braille library, as well as free medical services for the blind and their families" (p. 496).

To the "better educated" or successful blind, the lottery was little more than begging. However, most blind people viewed it as a positive alternative. In 1935, the Spanish Federation of the Blind agreed to pursue the national legitimization of their lotteries, but these efforts were engulfed by the political turmoil which led to the Spanish Civil War (1936-1939). From these historical developments and the political situation that developed in Spain in the latter days of the Civil War, the ONCE emerged.

BEGINNINGS OF THE ONCE

In 1938, in the midst of the civil war and "at a time when passions and opposing world views violently clashed, a group of young blind people, a handful of crazy visionaries, dared to conceive the idea that for the visually disabled it was a good moment to create a strategy that would allow them to progress toward a better future" (Zurita, 1994, p. 15). They wanted to see the situation of visually impaired Spaniards improved. Representatives of the blind argued persuasively that the new state would not be able to meet the welfare demands of the civilian and veteran blind (Garvía, 1995, p. 247).

One of the blind leaders was Javier Gutierrez de Tovar who, in October 1938, read a presentation in Braille during a national meeting of scholars concerned with public welfare issues. He argued for a program that would provide a secure economic base for blind people in Spain. For more than two hundred years, Spain had had national lotteries, and Tovar proposed that the organized blind people of Spain, be granted permission to run a legalized national lottery. The scholars at the conference agreed, and Tovar was among those presenting the recommendation to General Franco. On December 13, 1938, General Franco signed a decree establishing the Organización Nacional de Ciegos Españoles (ONCE). At age twenty-eight, Gutierrez de Tovar, a blind physical therapist, became its first leader.

The new group took advantage of the political opportunity afforded by the authoritarian regime, which was then consolidating its control over Spain. Just as the Chinese revolution later led to the creation of a comprehensive disabled people's organization for China (see Chapter 6), so too had the prevailing political climate of Spain resulted in a new unified organization. However, instead of a comprehensive organization for all disabled people, General Franco's decree dealt exclusively with the concerns of blind people. During the formative period of the ONCE, activities were conducted under general government supervision. Its purpose was to use existing resources as effectively as possible. "In effect, the government decree obliged all institutions of and for the blind existing at the time to disband as independent bodies and to merge assets and people into the new organization" (Zurita, 1994, p. 16). The national director was appointed by the government, and all visually impaired persons were required to be members of the new national organization.

Although under general government oversight, the ONCE was managed by blind people themselves and became the most important influence in Spain on their lives. First, one single organization managed all of the services and represented the interests of blind people to the state. Second, the revenues from the daily national lottery became the chief source of income for the ONCE and helped it become the largest employer of blind people in the country. Soon all blind children known to the organization were enrolled in schools and a high percentage of blind adults were employed.

A NEW OCCUPATION: FROM BEGGING TO SELLING LOTTERY TICKETS

The ONCE required large numbers of ticket sellers to create revenues sufficient for its ambitious education and social programs. Thousands of positions as lottery ticket sellers were created. This growth was seen as a mixed blessing within the ONCE's membership. The gradual movement towards "professionalizing" this occupation is well analyzed and documented in Professor Roberto Garvía's 1996 article, "The Professional Blind in Spain."

In the 1950s the leaders of the ONCE were not enthusiastic about creating jobs for blind people because, in their eyes, it resembled begging. They thought this reinforced the public stereotype that begging was the only kind of work blind people could do. This issue was a major area of contention within the ONCE during its first three decades. In the early days, leaders frequently had more formal education and occupations other than begging, for example, physiotherapy. They envisioned using the ONCE's money for vocational training and other forms of education that would enable blind people to be employed in various occupations throughout society. Even before the ONCE had been created the leadership was already divided over the economic future. Mr. Equerra, addressing the 1935 national assembly of the Federation argued:

> . . . Other friends of ours, in the minority, show themselves to be very alarmed at the idea that the lottery tickets might be implemented in a general manner over the entire country. They believe this implementation would have fatal consequences for the cultural and professional life of the Spanish blind. Who would think to study, to work, to toil, to move forward if the simple holding in one's hands a fistful of lottery tickets would solve his economic problems without any energy expenditure, without having to compete against anyone   and earning a daily wage that costs the seeing worker eight hours of exhausting labor? (Garvía, 1994, p. 22)

To alter the traditional stereotypes, the ONCE asked its vendors to dress presentably, use white canes and wear dark glasses. This was the first step in separating begging from blindness.

One way to destroy the stereotypes associated with begging was to create job training programs similar to those already existing in other European countries. Centers were established to train physical therapists, telephone operators, and factory workers. During this period the ONCE decided to accept partially sighted people as both members and employees. This expanded the available labor force and revenues were enhanced. However, the number of positions outside the lottery process was small; for the most part, lottery vending was the most common occupation. Up to the 1970s the ONCE had a candy wrapping factory. Most of the employees were women. When it closed, they were all employed in other ONCE's services.

The sale of lottery tickets did not meet the occupational aspirations of the better educated. Yet to many Spaniards, blind people had created their own problem. They had created a "lottery factory." The need for more revenue for more social programs required additional lottery vendors. A "ghetto" had been created by blind people for themselves: "By doing this, the blind have reinforced the social prejudices about their helplessness and incapacity, which explained their social isolation and lack of any other occupational prospect than the sale of their lottery tickets" (Garvía, 1996, pp. 500-501). Some viewed it as a shameful occupation, the only one the blind could do. Many blind people even regretted the changes that required them to give up begging.

GOAL DISPLACEMENT

During this period, Tovar continued his strong leadership of the ONCE. Garvía documents the gradual shift from the original goals of the ONCE to those that have become dominant during the past two decades: "Tovar's idea fundamentally was to apply all funds from the Second Quota to a welfare benefits system, not to the creation of factories, workshops or vocational schools" (p. 34). The Second Quota, masterminded by Tovar in 1943, provided for a larger percentage of revenues for the central organization which could be used for social and welfare benefits for the membership. Before this, only 12.5 percent of sales went to the central organization; it now became 32.5 percent. With these new funds there were sick leave and retirement benefits, as well as educational opportunities. Funds for international cooperation and special programs for people with other disabilities soon became available. In Tovar's words, "Do not doubt that by taking advantage of excessive sales [we are] going to ensure the well being of every blind man in his old age, in the case of disability, in illness and those numerous cases of defenselessness in which we find many of our children, wives and parents in the moment of our decease" (Garvía, 1994, p. 34). More lottery ticket sellers meant more general revenues, which grew so much that the ONCE can now provide the complete array of education and social welfare programs for its membership.

Two surveys during the 1970s found that lottery sellers did not view their occupations as negatively as did the "elites" of ONCE (Garvía, 1996, p. 501). They liked being economically independent and having a regular income. What could be done to improve the image of lottery sellers in the public eye? Two approaches always seemed to work: improving the work setting and increasing the level of compensation. In earlier decades, the ONCE was considered a charity and its workers volunteers, sometimes receiving compensation by being given lottery tickets. Now they were to be recognized as paid workers. In 1985, the ONCE introduced a five-day work week and clearly stated procedures for determining who received the most desirable vending locations. To this day, the ONCE lottery tickets are not sold on Saturdays or Sundays. They created a union and demanded higher salaries. In 1984, a new version of the lottery resulted in expanded sales and workers' salaries were raised by 77 percent.

> The new lottery was such a successful product that, at least during January 1984, buyers waited at street corners for the blind sellers to come, and a reselling market of lottery tickets even flourished. These unanticipated events showed the blind sellers that their customers did not buy their lottery tickets out of compassion, but because it was a competitive product in the gambling market. (Garvía, 1996, p. 502)

In their own eyes, they were no longer beggars but workers selling a popular product. However, those with more formal education continued to be concerned when some blind people working in various other occupations preferred to become ticket sellers. Salaries continued to improve, however, and the appearance of many vending locations was enhanced. Kiosks were built. Some began to think of themselves as "professionals." At present, instead of earning a living by begging, most ONCE workers earn twice the level of typical factory workers and have a lower unemployment rate. By 1988, 71 percent of the labor force of the ONCE sold lottery tickets, another 27 percent worked in other ONCE positions including education and rehabilitation services, while 2 percent worked in occupations outside the ONCE (Garvía, 1994, p. 25).

The ONCE's experience and success is unique. While many of their fellow blind in Europe and the United States were becoming clients of the welfare state, blind workers in Spain were being well paid and involved in one of Spain's most dynamic businesses. Gambling is extremely popular in Spain and a state sponsored lottery and other forms of gambling compete with the organization. ONCE's workers are employed in a widely recognized sector of the economy. In March, 1997, I interviewed several ONCE ticket sellers and observed others at their work. They were clearly proud of their organization and considered their employment as honorable and dignified as that of other occupations.

The political climate of Spain became more open in the 1960s and changes came to the ONCE as well. "The appointment as National Director of ONCE in 1959, of Ignacio Satrustegui, a prestigious entrepreneur who had lost his sight in the Civil War and who had been managing his own companies, brought some changes to the organization which mainly took the shape of a series of establishments set up for vocational training and basic rehabilitation" (Zurita, 1994, p. 17). ONCE now began to train people in an expanding array of occupations such as telephone operators, specialized factory workers and physiotherapists. Those employed in occupations outside the ONCE continued to grow in number. However, rather than working in a factory, many preferred selling lottery tickets within the ONCE because it resulted in a larger income with less difficult work (Burns, 1989, p. 31).

To the pleasure of many, Spain experienced a rapid transition towards a more democratic government and the new generation of younger blind people wanted the same for the ONCE. Change came, but not without resistance from the older generation within. "They thought that these young agitators who were claiming freedom and democracy were going to destroy that great work they had built with the sacrifice of so many people over many years" (Zurita, 1994, p. 17). In 1981, a government decree amended the original charter, incorporating democratic reforms. Since 1981, the ONCE has been governed by fifteen blind people who comprise its General Council, elected every four years by a process which enfranchises all adult members. The first new generation of leaders was installed with the 1982 election. "Nearly all of them were under the age of thirty. Some had university educations, others had gained their experience in the school of life that was the sale of the lottery tickets on the streets of many cities in Spain, at times done in quite harsh conditions" (Zurita, 1994, p. 17). In 1982, Antonio Vicente Mosquete became the leader of the new democratic ONCE. The resulting reforms included a streamlined lottery process which made it more attractive to the purchasers of tickets. Enhanced revenue growth resulted. In fact, sales soon doubled and provided a stronger economic base for future development. During the period 1984-1994, the ONCE's revenues increased eightfold.

One of the ONCE's major accomplishments is a 95 percent employment rate for blind people, surely the highest percentage of blind people employed in the labor force of any country in the world.

"In absolute figures, we can say that 14,384 blind and partially sighted people are employed as vendors of ONCE's lottery, and they receive monthly salaries that are notably higher than the average salary of Spanish workers" (Zurita, 1994, p. 18). In addition to all of the benefits afforded by the ONCE, lottery vendors are also eligible to participate in Spain's Social Security system. Some vendors still sell tickets on the streets, but more recently and more commonly lottery tickets are sold at vending stands located in train stations, airports, department stores, and many public places.

Other than in lottery sales and administration, more than one thousand additional blind workers have well-paying positions in services and programs supported by the ONCE. The ONCE finances two main book production centers: Centro Bibliográfico y Cultural in Madrid and Centro de Producción Bibliográfica in Barcelona. Apart from these, there are many decentralized book production units. In addition, the ONCE supports a museum, several schools, rehabilitation centers, and home-based rehabilitation services. In these areas and in the management of the ONCE, almost all of the leadership positions are occupied by people who are blind.

EXPANDING THE ONCE'S PROGRAM FOR PEOPLE WITH PHYSICAL DISABILITIES

In 1987, the ONCE's programs expanded in a new and important direction for people with disabilities in Spain. A foundation was established, The Fundación ONCE, and 3 percent of the organization's revenues were dedicated to provide services to people with physical limitations other than blindness. "As a consequence of its policy of solidarity, it is able to finance the activities of the ONCE foundation for promoting employment and for the elimination of all types of obstacles for other collective groups of disabled persons" (An Introduction to ONCE, 1994, p.1). Factories and other enterprises were purchased to provide employment, and as of 1994, seven thousand nonblind individuals with some form of physical disability were employed as lottery vendors. Others were employed in several different ONCE-related enterprises.

With the passage of a decade, the ONCE looks back to the beginning of this new program and refers to it as "solidarity." However, the situation was more complicated in the decade leading to 1987. The competition for gaming revenues was intense and the legal lotteries, such as the ONCE, did not like the "underground competition." "An especially notorious example of this situation is the company PRODIECU, S.A., which has been operating in the wagering market without a single administrative license or authorisation, the social justification for this situation being the company's alleged pro-handicapped policy" (de Lorenzo Garcia, 1987, p. 24). PRODIECU, a lottery run for people with disabilities other than blindness, provided stiff competition to the ONCE.

> PRODIECU's lottery was sold by approximately 7,000 physically disabled people who had taken inspiration from the success of the lottery of the blind and decided to launch their own. This lottery was not only a commercial threat to ONCE, but also put into question its institutional privilege which was (and still is) based on the exclusive right of the blind to operate in the gaming market. (Garvía, 1996, p. 503)

The government was reluctant to enforce laws against an illegal lottery which was providing so many employment opportunities for handicapped people. The ONCE vendors confronted daily competition on many street corners from PRODIECU's vendors. As in the United States and most European countries, blind people had strong national organizations long before other disability groups. To avoid harmful competition and possible threats to its monopoly in the national political arena, the ONCE had to come to terms with PRODIECU. PRODIECU's former members now work in the ONCE and the ONCE's social and educational programs are available to all disability groups.

Coming to terms does not do justice to the intense economic and political competition the ONCE confronted during this period. With so much money involved, it was inevitable that other disability groups and organizations of older people should seek a way to access lottery revenues. The ONCE handled this competition in a way that demonstrates the political resourcefulness and the economic skills of its leadership.

The ONCE's first strategy was to divide and conquer: to employ some people with disabilities other than blindness in order to blunt the charge that other disability groups should have access to the same opportunities as ONCE's membership. Those privileged to now be ONCE ticket sellers became staunch supporters of the ONCE. "The second strategy consisted of promoting the creation of a national organization of the physically disabled and making it financially dependent on ONCE's resources in order to control its demands" (Garvía, 1995, p. 248). The ONCE wanted to provide services sufficient to ensure the cooperation of disability groups, but it wanted to control the cost of this cooperation. The ONCE could not utilize the state as an ally; public officials would have difficulty justifying a legal monopoly for the blind to the exclusion of other disability groups.

During the period of 1970-1986, the government issued decrees in response to the demands of disabled people and other advocacy groups such as parents with disabled children. These included calls for pensions, better employment opportunities, and the removal of architectural barriers. The government's finances were so restricted that these policies were largely unfunded. One answer was the previously mentioned illegal company, PRODIECU. Not only was it not legally chartered, but it was managed by nonhandicapped people, doubtless to their considerable economic benefit. As PRODIECU spread across Spain, its leadership was laying the cornerstone for the claim that another ONCE-type national organization should be recognized by the government.

In 1977, an umbrella organization was created to broadly represent the interests of various disability groups: Coordinadora Estatal de Minusvalidos Fisicos (CEMFE). CEMFE, in the midst of a struggle for survival, decided not to support the efforts of other disability groups for a new lottery. It criticized PRODIECU, alleging that handicapped people were being exploited by the non-handicapped who managed PRODIECU. By criticizing other disability groups and refusing to support demands for a new lottery, it risked losing its political base among people with disabilities. However, this stance gave CEMFE the chance to present itself as a responsible and law-abiding organization; through moderation and bargaining it would advance the cause through disabled people.

Naturally, ONCE was sympathetic to the only national organization of disabled people that did not threaten its monopoly. "After repeatedly and publicly denouncing PRODIECU as a company which profited from the hardships of the physically disabled, CEMFE received economic and administrative support from ONCE" (Garvía, 1995, p.

251). When CEMFE used ONCE's funds to start programs for disabled people, it was recapturing its natural political base. The ONCE announced it wished to employ 1,000 physically disabled and asked CEMFE to participate in this selection process. The ONCE was funded and thus cooperating with a major disability organization that did not challenge its monopoly.

However, PRODIECU was using 7,000 disabled people to sell illegal lottery tickets, and this hurt both the ONCE and the state run lottery. The government could not easily crack down on PRODIECU and put so many people out of work. At the same time, neither the government nor the ONCE wanted another legal lottery. Many ordinary citizens, learning about this conflict through the public media, felt sympathy for the various disability groups -- why were the blind so special?

The ONCE leadership developed a successful strategy: the ONCE would hire an additional 7,000 disabled lottery ticket sellers, which would relieve the political pressure on it to crack down on the non-handicapped people who profited from PRODIECU. The strategy worked. "In short, ONCE's strategy was to defeat PRODIECU in the political arena (and not in the market arena); to strengthen CEMFE and control the future demands of the physically disabled; and to make the state pay for it" (Garvía, 1995, p. 252).

As a compromise with the state, the ONCE agreed to set aside a small percentage of its revenues into a special trust to provide social services for disability groups other than the blind. Now the ONCE was helping the state by funding social programs for the otherwise disabled and providing employment for more than 7,000 disabled people.

> In order to carry out its new welfare role, ONCE created Fundacion ONCE, honoring its old proposal to set up a solidarity fund in exchange for the dismantling previously supported and devised by the state. There are now administered by the blind, in close collaboration with the interest organizations of the physically disabled (COCEMFE, previously CEMFE), the deaf-mute (CNSE) and representatives of the mentally handicapped (FIAPAS). (Garvía, 1995, p. 254)

Under this new foundation, cooperation between the ONCE and other disability groups continued to improve. The ONCE did keep political control of the foundation's Board of Directors, and its resources were used to everyone's advantage. In its first year of operation, the Foundation created more than 1,000 new jobs for disabled people. In contrast, the state, had created only 300 jobs in the previous three years through its affirmative action policies. Thus, the ONCE emerged from two decades of intense competition and political struggle with both its corporate structure and lottery monopoly intact. It had eliminated most of its competition and become a significant provider for the social programs of other disability groups. No longer could public officials or rival groups criticize it for being a lottery only for the blind.

EXPANDING THE ONCE'S BUSINESS INTERESTS

Between 1988 and 1992 the ONCE broadened its economic base by purchasing part interest, and frequently, controlling interest, in revenue producing enterprises other than the lottery. In most cases, blind people held management positions in these ONCE owned undertakings. During this period, the General Director of the ONCE, Miguel Duran, received international attention when he became chairman of one of Spain's largest telecommunication companies. "Miguel Duran led, to a large extent, this aggressive policy of participating in the economic life of the country and owing to his great personal charm and extraordinary gift for communication, he has become a very popular public figure" (Zurita, 1994, p. 19).

Today, the ONCE leadership continues to diversify in additional sectors of the economy. For example, in 1996 "ONCE purchased a significant interest in a Five Star luxury complex on the Isle of Margarita, a Caribbean island belonging to Venezuela" (Reuters, December 17, 1996). Also, "Union des Assurances de Paris (VAP), Paris has signed an agreement with Organización Nacional de Ciegos Españoles (ONCE), the financially powerful organization for the blind which controls the distribution of lottery tickets, to sell a range of insurance policies" (*Financial Times*, February 14, 1992). In 1993 the *Institutional Investor* newspaper also reported:

Organizacion Nacional de Ciegos Españoles the cash-rich Spanish association for the blind, earns 300 billion pesetas ($3 billion) from lotteries a year, and boasts a huge investment portfolio of pesetas as 150 billion plus. So ambitious

director, Miguel Duran, who has taken the charity into almost every sector of
the Spanish economy and built up a reputation as an aggressive corporate
raider and arbitrageur, was one of the most courted but feared players on
Madrid's thriving bolsa. (p. 2)

The ONCE's economic adversity and rapid growth is summarized
in a June 8, 1991, newspaper article from *The Independent of London*:

Don't be deceived by the blind man selling lottery tickets on any Spanish street
corner. Behind him is one of the most impressive financial empires in the country, growing rapidly and set on a collision course with the government. The
Organizacion Nacional de Ciegos Españoles (ONCE) has interests in the construction industry, in Spain's largest bank, Banco Bilbao Vizcaya, and in
supermarket companies and venture capital firms. It is planning to develop a
holiday resort for the blind on an island off the coast of Venezuela, owns a
newspaper and radio station, and has a share in a new commercial television
station. It sponsors a successful cycling team. Yet, less than a decade ago,
ONCE was virtually bankrupt. (p.4)

From manufacturing to insurance to television to radio stations to construction, and so forth, the ONCE's economic diversification helps
provide more varied work opportunities for its members and places its
finances on a broader base.

BLIND PEOPLE TAKING CARE OF THEMSELVES

One consequence of the ONCE's employment of so many blind
workers is that the Spanish citizens regularly encounter blind people
at a greater rate than in any other nation. Also, the ONCE maintains
constant communication with the public through print and radio and
television commercials about the lottery and the services which lottery
revenues help fund. Most services for blind people, and now some services for people with other disabilities, are paid for, not by public tax-
ation, but by lottery revenues in which the citizenry participates vol-
untarily. The ONCE is not seen as a welfare program. "So far as the
public at large is concerned, ONCE, as compared to ten of the most
representative humanitarian institutions in Spain, was known to nearly all those surveyed (99%), and its social work was rated highly"
(Gonzalez, 1994, p. 32).

There has been another important consequence for blind people as a result of the economic success of the ONCE: "The blindness/poverty connection has definitely vanished from the minds of the public in general, and from social and economic agents in particular. The ONCE is admired and respected, and often bankers and entrepreneurs are found courting its directors in an attempt to gain their favor" (Zurita, 1994, p. 20).

THE ONCE'S PROGRAM

The ONCE has developed a holistic approach to providing education and rehabilitation services to its members:

> Our services are conceived on the basis of an integral view of the individual, making it a unique model among organizations for the disabled. In order to do this, the organization has an important network composed of thirty-three centers where basic services are offered and eleven specialized centers that attend to the principal needs of more than fifty thousand members. (An Introduction to ONCE, 1994, p. 2)

The social service department of the ONCE coordinates the work of more than 1,100 specialists providing services to its members.

In 1996, the ONCE's budget provided the following support for its different types of programs: Education–8,622,000 pesetas ($6,122,000); Professional Training and Rehabilitation–4,255,000 pesetas ($3,021,000); Activities Related to Technical Devices and Complementary Services–7,565,000 pesetas ($5,371,000); Cultural and Recreational Activities–4,452,000 pesetas ($3,161,000). These numbers are quoted in pesetas with the approximate April 1997 U.S. dollar value in brackets (An Introduction to ONCE, 1994, p. 2).

Membership in the ONCE is open to blind and visually impaired Spanish citizens who are screened for eligibility by an ophthalmologist provided by the ONCE. Membership is free; those interested can contact one of the more than three hundred ONCE centers distributed throughout the country, where information and counseling are provided. Membership as of March 31, 1997 totaled 52,431.

The membership can receive appropriate assistance from a wide array of the ONCE services. These include prevention of blindness programs, training to facilitate independent living, support for individuals with disabilities in addition to blindness, and vocational placement in addition to lottery sales and the management and monitoring of financial assistance to the ONCE members:

> Young, visually impaired people wishing to undertake vocational training can attend ordinary centers or the ONCE Educational Centers in Madrid, Barcelona and Seville, in which they can study the following subjects: monographic courses in telephony, stenotyping, piano tuning, etc.; secretarial studies, telematics, business management, languages, radiophonics, etc. Likewise, the ONCE has a Physiotherapy School in Madrid for training in this field. Young people wishing to study other university courses have the support of the Basic Care Teams. (Lazaro, 1993, p. 12)

Rehabilitation services are tailored to the needs of the individual, including particular programs for those with different levels of visual loss. For example, specialists provide everything from orientation and mobility training to instruction in the use of low vision aids. Emphasis is placed on the acquisition of skills to heighten the individual's personal autonomy. "Depending on the individual characteristics and situation of the person to be rehabilitated, the various alternative kinds of care are as follows: Basic Care Teams; Rehabilitation Units (Madrid and Seville); Castel Arnau Rehabilitation Centre; Educational Resource Centers" (Guide to ONCE, p. 34). ONCE has continued to add new programs for special needs groups within its membership. For example, there is now a guide dog training facility, a program for people with diabetes, home health care and drug rehabilitation services. "Specialized services are also provided for senior citizens including apartments and other lodgings, day care centers, recreational interest group activities and other services to promote independent living" (Lazaro, 1993, pp. 5-8).

Financial aid is also provided to support the client's involvement in the ONCE's programs. First, pensions are designed to cover disabilities for individuals between the ages of eighteen and sixty-five, and old age pensions for those over sixty-five. Second, four types of financial aid are provided: nonperiodic, temporary aid to families, aid to third parties and other special aid. Finally, technical aid includes support to agencies or organizations providing assistance to the ONCE members. For example, technical assistance is given to residential schools, teachers of blind students in ordinary schools, providers of in-home care, and workers conducting vocational training for the ONCE members.

The ONCE also provides support to individuals not eligible, for whatever reason, to participate in Spain's social security system. This category includes the multiply-disabled, senior citizens and others not eligible for the state sponsored social security system. For its multi-handicapped members, the ONCE provides information and counseling, independent living, education and financial aid, and contemplates supportive collaboration with other entities and institutions (INSERSO), regional governments, associations, private centers and so forth) specializing in handicaps concurrent with visual impairment, so as to provide the best and most complete service possible (An Introduction to ONCE).

In particular, the ONCE's services for the elderly focus on independent living. The programs include home care, house cleaning, aid in personal hygiene, specialized counseling, and residential adaptations necessary for independent living. Assistance in locating, and, if necessary, subsidizing housing is also provided. Recreational and leisure activities in group settings and in the home are also made available. In addition, the ONCE cooperates with other public and private agencies, providing services to people with various types of substance addictions, diabetes, and blind persons who are also deaf. In July, 1997, the ONCE sponsored a European conference for the deafblind and those who provide educational and rehabilitation service to them. Deafblind people tend to think that their disability is not an addition of blindness and deafness, but it is a disability on its own. They have agreed, and the Spaniards follow this habit that the word *deafblind* should be written without a hyphen separation in it.

To help its members find employment, the ONCE offers financial aid to permit appropriate training for job placement, counseling for those having difficulty in adjusting to their work setting, training courses in specialized fields such as computer work, low interest loans to permit self employment opportunities, and education to help employers recognize the advantages of hiring blind workers. The ONCE provides several kinds of support for both schools, teachers and blind students themselves. The philosophy emphasizes integration into the community, but the ONCE recognizes the importance of specialized services necessary for the education of blind students. "It is believed that the best way of rehabilitating children is through the highest possible degree of integration into the educational system, as this constitutes the basis of the child's organizational and environmental support" (Martinez Henarejos, 1989, p. 13). This is illustrated by excerpts from a June 27, 1995 article which appeared in the *Manchester Guardian* entitled, "Special Touch in Spain."

> Miriam is a blind student who studies at her local school in Barcelona, thanks to the assistance provided by specialists from the Joan Amades Centre. Joan Amades (1890-1959), was a blind writer who wrote about folklore in Catalonia. In Spain, the story of the integration of blind and visually handicapped stu dents within local schools started nine years ago at the Centre, also based in Barcelona. "It was when we demonstrated the benefits of integrated education and the importance of being surrounded by family and friends in your own neighbourhood," explains Joan J. Torres, the school's director, who is also blind.
>
> Miriam Galan was four when her parents finally admitted that she had problems with her sight and took her to the Centre. In her school Miriam received a normal education. In the Joan Amades Centre she acquires the techniques to enable her to learn and to be as independent as possible in everyday life.

The ONCE facilitates "mainstreaming" in several different ways, appropriate to the needs of individual students. A student might spend one day a week at a ONCE-sponsored center, learning skills leading to independent living. Involvement in residential schools usually decreases as a child progresses educationally. A specialist from the ONCE may visit a student, such as Miriam, to provide instruction, to help support her progress in regular activities. Through this specialist educational material can be made available in Braille in a timely manner and/or the student may continue to progress with computers having electronic speech capability. While working with the regular classroom teacher, the child's parents and student, the ONCE specialist may involve other professionals—again provided through the ONCE. Throughout Spain local school teachers can rely on special education assistance from the ONCE and the blind student, and the student's family can be confident that any assistance provided will demonstrate a positive philosophy about blindness, and about the potential of blind students to compete in terms of equality.

As of May 1997, the Department of Education reports the ONCE is involved in the education of 6,319 children; of these, 642 attended the ONCE centers full time and the rest were enrolled in regular public schools. The five educational resource centers are located in the following cities: Madrid, Barcelona, Seville, Alicante, and Pontevedra. The philosophy includes involving the child's family in the education process. The earliest detection of blindness and the earliest detection of diseases in progress are stressed (Lazaro, 1993, p. 10).

INTERNATIONAL COOPERATION

In Chapter 2, I described some aspects of the influence of international government organizations on services for the blind. For the most part, these organizations insist upon generalized, community-based approaches to rehabilitation. However, many within the organized blind movement argue that specialized services that provide skills for literacy, mobility and independent living are essential to the education and rehabilitation of blind children and adults.

In Chapter 5, I described international cooperation affecting blind people in several African nations. In general, international cooperation of blindness agencies follows old patterns of colonial domination. For example, programs from the United Kingdom are more likely to be transposed to former English speaking colonies. Sometimes, problems arise while grafting programs from the outside on to indigenous cultural traditions.

Spain has a distinct cultural and historical relationship with almost all countries in Latin America. The ONCE has the economic resources and the willingness to provide economic support and other services to these Latin American nations. Organizations of blind people in other countries sometimes share their economic resources, expressing solidarity with other blind people in less economically developed countries. However, no nation comes even close to the level of economic resources which the ONCE makes available for international cooperation.

In addition to aid for specific countries, since 1984 the ONCE has provided significant levels of support to the World Blind Union (WBU). The costs of the office of the Secretary General of the World Blind Union, located in Madrid, is essentially underwritten by the ONCE. This is currently under the able leadership of Pedro Zurita, current Secretary General. Mr. Zurita has been re-elected three times by the membership of the World Blind Union.

The following comes from an article by Kepa Conde Zabala entitled, "Funding Aid for Latin America: ONCE/ULAC Cooperation Fund with Ibero-America, Twelve Years of Assistance," which appeared in the July, 1996, issue of *The World Blind* (pp. 17-18). This summarizes the ONCE's international cooperation with and economic support of more than 1,000 organizations and programs in Central and South America. Zabala notes that although ONCE supports over 1,000 organizations for the blind, there are limits to what this group can do. Rafael Mondaca, Chairman of the ONCE General Council's Commission on International Relations, feels that "these organizations must make every effort to obtain support to cofinance their projects, reduce their dependence on international NGOs and seek resources in their communities, rather than expecting support from the ONCE alone. Besides empowering their associations of the blind and becoming truly representative, these organizations must realize that their future is at stake unless they are able to raise funds from other resources" (p. 17).

According to Mondaca, the ONCE has financed Latin American blind people because this support represents "solidarity towards a region that is very dear to our hearts." However, the support has taken different forms in succeeding years. Early on, it consisted of Braille and talking books, financing for professional development, and blindness prevention opportunities. In 1984, an effort was made to systematize support within ONCE's General Council's founding charter. The Fund was "intended to contribute to the financing of cooperation programs in the fields of welfare and care for visually disabled people" (p. 17). In 1986, the Fund was placed under the umbrella of the World Blind Union (WBU). In 1988, a new period began where not only did the Fund receive UNUM checks but also received donations in the form of materials from the ONCE Aids and Devices for the Blind Unit (UTT). In 1989, the ONCE created a school kit that contained basic materials needed by blind pupils.

In that same year, a new approach was taken. The ONCE/ULAC Cooperation Fund asked that organizations needing assistance fill out annual applications describing their specific needs with explanations for the needs. The call for applications stated "we must continue to redouble our efforts to provide children and young adults access to the tools they need to study; to ensure men and women rehabilitation and paid employment; to enable our teachers to acquire greater expertise;

in short, to guarantee that everyone is in a position to exercise their rights and equal opportunities to fully participate in society" (p. 18). Applications are circulated to associations and organizations of and for the blind (individuals are not eligible) in January of each year. In October, the commission decides which projects will be funded. The Fund is in contact with 1,039 institutions throughout Latin America: "206 in Argentina, 33 in Bolivia, 337 in Brazil, 88 in Colombia, 12 in Costa Rica, 21 in Cuba, 50 in Chile, 12 in the Dominican Republic, 47 in Ecuador, 6 in El Salvador, 9 in Guatemala, 10 in Honduras, 63 in Mexico, 12 in Nicaragua, 9 in Panama, 7 in Paraguay, 61 in Peru, 24 in Uruguay and 28 in Venezuela. It also cooperates with Puerto Rico and, on occasion, with Haiti" (p. 18).

The applications received in 1996 can be classified in eight categories: "208 projects for teaching materials, 242 for furtherance of Braille and talking books, 322 for services, 79 for job placement, 4 for production of aids and devices, 64 for meetings and courses, 29 for organizational expenses and 49 for sports" (p. 18), totaling 997. Of these, the Commission approved 332 (33.3%).

In the first twelve years, the Fund experienced certain difficulties such as a constant change in the management of the governing body, little government involvement, too many organizations of and for the blind, tendencies to atomize efforts, and difficulties in obtaining import licenses. However, there were also accomplishments. There was a recognition for the need for unity, cooperation with NGOs in the area, the introduction and use of high technology equipment, a greater ability of aids and devices for the blind, and a rise in paid employment. There were also specific types of assistance provided such as teaching materials and equipment for the schools, the furtherance of Braille and talking books, services helping with early intervention and visual rehabilitation, help with job placement, the production of equipment needed by the blind, training for those educating the blind and leading organizations assisting the blind, and the promotion of organizations for the blind.

SUMMARY

In fewer than sixty years, most blind people in Spain are no longer among the poorest citizens; they are relatively prosperous. The unemployment rate for blind people is much lower than the unemployment rate in the national labor force. The minimum wage for entry level blind workers in the ONCE is more than two times the national minimum wage. The ONCE is controlled by blind people themselves through democratically-elected leaders. The ONCE employs and controls the people who provide special education and rehabilitation services to its members. It provides welfare and other benefits for those who are unable to work or who are retired. It provides employment and social programs for people with disabilities other than blindness. It has acquired a wide array of economic enterprises to broaden its economic base; the ONCE does not depend entirely upon lottery revenues. Through its advertising and public relation efforts the ONCE is widely recognized and widely acclaimed throughout Spain. It has largely eliminated from Spanish culture the long-standing tradition that associated blindness with begging. Most ONCE workers are proud of their occupations and proud of their organization. They share some of their wealth through international cooperation with the World Blind Union and provide significant amounts of money to assist organizations of blind people in Latin America. In Spain, blind people are not clients of the welfare state, as is the case, in varying degrees, in other European nations and other societies around the world. Amidst all these accomplishments, are there still problems to be solved within the ONCE?

As we have noted in this chapter, many of the ONCE's early leaders were better educated than most blind people in Spain at that time. They envisioned an organization that would have the money to provide education and other opportunities so that blind people could work in occupations throughout society along side the rest of the labor force. Some felt that selling lottery tickets was not much better than begging, and that it would reinforce the stereotype that blind people can do only the simplest kinds of tasks. Although gambling is an old tradition in Spain, some question the economic significance of building so many employment opportunities on a lottery, which is not economically productive and which transfers funds from one group of citizens to another. Only a few win big; the real winner is the ONCE and its members. Without empirical evidence, some say that the poorer people of Spain primarily support the ONCE because the affluent, it is alleged, participate less in the lottery.

Others criticize the ONCE for becoming too economically and politically powerful. Why should a lottery run solely by blind people be allowed to be the base of what has become one of the top ten economic enterprises in Spain? Has the ONCE become too powerful? Why should the state run lottery have to put up with this competition? Is it proper for the ONCE to own more than two hundred radio stations as well as other media outlets, particularly when these are used to publicize the ONCE's lottery? Is it, somehow, wrong for the blind people of Spain to live in what might be called a "gilded ghetto"?

How might an outsider respond to these questions and criticisms? Let us first look at the ONCE's success in the business and financial world. In the free market of the Spanish economy, successful businesses are normally applauded and appreciated for their success and contributions to the Spanish economy. Would the ONCE's expanded business activities be criticized if they were the activities of "ordinary" people? Probably not. Yet, the success of the ONCE relieves the state of the high level of public funding required for special education and rehabilitation and social welfare services typical in other European and most industrial societies.

Second, we can examine the issue of gambling as a basis for employing blind people. Gambling, particularly in the form of lotteries, is quite common in Spain and predates by at least one hundred years the establishment of the ONCE. It is an acceptable form of recreation in Spain. When I tried to explain the apparent reason why some states in the United States refuse lotteries through elections, on the grounds that gambling is immoral or we should not encourage people to think of getting something for no effort, the ONCE ticket sellers I talked with only laughed. Most ONCE members simply reflect the widely held idea in Spain that lotteries are acceptable forms of entertainment and economic opportunity. In selling lottery tickets, they are doing the very same kind of work as their competitors in the state run lottery. People are not buying tickets out of pity or for charitable reasons, but for the opportunity to win money,—as they do in the state lottery.

Third, what can an outsider say about the "gilded ghetto"—the concern on the part of some that only 2 percent of Spain's blind labor force works outside the ONCE? Remember, in 1988, 71 percent of the ONCE's members sold lottery tickets while another 27 percent worked in administrative and other jobs within the ONCE. This is the more complicated issue to me. In the United States, most organizations of blind people fight for employment opportunities in the general labor force. The only alternatives are working in sheltered workshops or becoming dependent clients of the welfare state.

We can get an additional perspective on this issue by looking at the experience of another nation which is both historically and culturally related to Spain and which has received some assistance through the ONCE's international programs. Costa Rica, like other Latin American countries, presents a bleak prospect for the competitive employment of blind people. While 5 percent of Spain's blind work force is unemployed, in most parts of Latin America only 5 percent of blind people have jobs. This is so in Costa Rica, a country that is renowned for its political stability, traditions of democracy, and gradually improving economy. "In Costa Rica, blind people are mostly underemployed in jobs much beneath their skills and educational level and this and the institutions created to ensure their welfare have no clear policies regarding placement opportunities" (Sancho Alvarez, 1996, p. 31). Yet, Costa Rica has strong policies to protect the ordinary worker. Its national constitution includes the following provisions:

> Article 33: All men are equal under law and no discrimination contrary to human dignity shall be tolerated,
>
> Article 56: All individuals have the right and social obligation to work. The state must endeavor to ensure everyone honest, useful and duly remunerated employment and shall prevent the establishment of conditions that impair human freedom or dignity, and work that degrades human beings to the status of mere merchandise. (Sancho Alvarez, 1996, p. 31)

Costa Rica has the legal framework in place to assure equal opportunity. In fact, some of its blind citizens are employed as lawyers, school teachers, and as owners and workers in small businesses, but these are the exceptions.

Consider the same issue of employment in the United States. A small percentage of blind people, of whom I am one, have achieved employment in ordinary positions where one is judged by performance. However, I have never seen the unemployment rate of blind people in the United States drop below 70 percent and it is sometimes estimated to be as high as 85 percent. This, in spite of more than seventy years and billions of dollars of federal and state government support for vocational rehabilitation services. Affirmative Action programs, the Americans With Disabilities Act, and efforts to educate employers about the ability of blind workers have not yet made a significant dent on the high unemployment and underemployment rate. Thus, many blind Americans have no choice but to become dependent clients of the welfare state. From innumerable conversations, I know how difficult it is for most blind people in free market societies to find competitive employment. Most want to work, support themselves and be free of the welfare stigma associated with publicly-supported programs.

Having described the situation of blind people in Costa Rica and the United States, how can I condemn the ONCE for providing high levels of well paid employment? Should this success be disparaged because only a small percentage of the ONCE's members work outside the organization? I suspect that most blind people in most countries in the world would be very happy to be members of an organization like the ONCE. In a perfect world, it would be a desirable goal for blind people to be employed in most occupations throughout the labor force. In the real world of today, they confront competitive employment as the exception and the welfare state as the norm. That situation may some day change.

It will be difficult for the blind people of any country to create a business and organization like the ONCE. However, one should not rule out the possibility of employment opportunities through self-run organizations. In particular, they are a more likely possibility in countries experiencing rapid economic development.

Finally, there are several features of the ONCE that would be interesting for sociologists to study. What are the patterns of mobility within the ONCE? Do the better educated individuals disproportionally occupy more desirable positions? Do blind people from poor families have equal opportunities for improving their position in the ONCE? Does membership in the ONCE mean that their social networks operate primarily within the organization as compared to, for example, blind people in England or France? Is the conflict between professional educators and rehabilitation workers minimized in the ONCE because they are all employed by the ONCE? This has been a significant problem in the United States, but to my knowledge no one has studied this issue in an organization controlled by blind people themselves. Is blindness considered to be such a horrible fate in a country where blind workers are well employed and earn above average salaries? Would differences in self-pride and self concept be significant for the typical member of the ONCE and the typical welfare client of comparably industrialized societies? Finally, is gender an issue in the ONCE? These are only a few of the questions that have occurred to me since I have learned about this organization, an organization for which I have enormous respect.

BIBLIOGRAPHY

Albrecht, G. 1992. *The Disability Business: Rehabilitation in America.*Walnut Creek, CA: Sage.

Alvarez, R. 1996. Overview of the Employment Situation in Costa Rica. *The World Blind*, No. 13, July.

American Association of Workers for the Blind (AAWB) Proceedings. 1935. Committee Report.

An Introduction to the ONCE. Published by ONCE, printed in Madrid by Industria Gráfcia Altair, SA. p. 1.

Anonymous. 1990. The Blind in Zambia. *The World Blind*, No. 3, July-December, pp. 16 - 19.

Anonymous. 1996. Tuning in on Africa. *The World Blind.* July, No. 13, p. 12.

Barton, I. 1991. Disability and the Necessity for a Socio-Political Perspective. *The Monograph*, #51, pp. 1-14.

Bentzen, B. L. and Barlow, J. M. 1995. Impact of Curb Ramps on the Safety of Persons Who Are Blind. *Journal of Visual Impairment and Blindness.* 89(4), pp. 319-328.

Billington, J. & Karlsson, G. 1997. Body Experiences of Persons Who Are Congenitally Blind: A Phenomenological Psychological Study. *Journal of Visual Impairment and Blindness.* March - April, Volume 91, Number 2, p. 15.

Bruce, P. 1991. Spanish Charity Locks Horns with Ministry over Lottery–Spain. *The Financial Times,* June 4. London.

Buckley, S. 1997. Africa's Disabled Organize to Fend Off Discrimination of Wheel Chairs: Finding Ways Into Offices, Legislatures. *Washington Post Foreign Service.* June 3.

Burgess, J. 1928. *The Guilds of Peking.* New York: Columbia University Press.

Burns, T. 1989. ONCE in the Eye of the Hurricane. *Financial Times Limited,* London.

Busk, P. L. & Marascvilo, L. A. 1992. Statistical Analysis in Single-Case Research: Issues, Procedures and Recommendations with Applications to Multiple Behaviors in *Single-Case Research Design and Analysis: New Directions for Psychology and Education.* (Eds.) Kocetochwill, T. and Levin, J. Lawrence Erlbaum Associates, New Jersey.

Chan, G. 1996. Regional Cooperation–A Key to Mutual Enhancement and Mutual Benefit. *The Educator*, pp. 19-23.

Clemens, S. 1910. *Mark Twain's Speeches.* New York and London: Harper and Brothers.

Coleman, D. M. 1947. *A History of the Nashville Workshop for the Blind: 1918-1946.* Department of Public Welfare, Nashville, Tennessee. Available from the library at the National Center for the Blind, 1800 Johnson Street, Baltimore, Maryland.

de Lorenzo Garcia, R. 1987. The Granting of Lottery Concession as a Source of Financing Social Services for the Visually Handicapped and as a Major Means of Employment. Paper presented at International Conference on Social Legislation Concerning the Rights of the Blind and the Visually Handicapped in Various European Countries. September.

Deshen, S. 1992. *Blind People: The Private and Public Life of Sightless Israelis.* New York: State University of New York Press.

Duff-Brown, B. 1995. Taming the Lion's Look; World Health Agency Trying to Stop River Blindness. *Los Angeles Times,* The Times Mirror Company.

Eckery, L. 1991. What Color is the Sun? Published in *What Color is the Sun,* ed. by Kenneth Jernigan. Published at the National Federation of the Blind, Baltimore, Maryland.

Education of the Handicapped in China. 1989. Disabilities in China. Beijing: The Association for the Handicapped, February.

Education of the Handicapped in China. 1989. Disabilities in China. Beijing: The Association for the Handicapped, October.

Eisenstadt, S. N. 1964. *From Generation to Generation.* London: The Free Press of Glencoe, Collier-MacMillan Limited.

Fairbank, J. 1986. *The Great Revolution: 1800-1985.* New York: Harper & Row.

Fairbank, J. & Reischaver, E. 1989. *China: Tradition and Transformation.* Boston: Houghton-Mifflin.

Farrell, G. 1956. *The Story of Blindness.* Cambridge, MA: Harvard University Press.

Feagin, R., Orum,. M., & Sjoberg,. (eds). 1991. *A Case for the Case Study.*Chapel Hill, NC: University of North Carolina Press.

Fefoame, G. 1996. Issues Affecting Blind Women in the Rehabilitation Process. Paper presented at the African Forum. Published in African Forum Proceedings, World Blind Union Institutional Development Project, Watertown, Massachusetts.

Ferrell, K. A. 1984. A Second Look at Sensory Aids in Early Childhood. *Education of the Visually Handicapped.* 16, pp. 83-101.

French, R. S. 1932. *From Homer to Helen Keller.* New York: American Foundation for the Blind.

Fryer, G. 1942. Report on Work for the Blind in China: 1931-1941. *Outlook for the Blind and the Teachers Forum.* June, 36: 3.

Garmezy, N. 1982. The Case for Single Case in Research in *Single-Case Research Designs: Methods for Clinical and Applied Settings.* (Eds.) H. Kazdin and A. Hussain Tuma. New York: Oxford University Press.

Garvia, R. 1994. "Revisiting Rationality in Organization: The Case of the Spanish Organization of the Blind." Working Paper Series #55. Cambridge, MA: Center for European Studies.

Garvia, R. 1995. Corporation, Public Policy and Welfare: The Case of the Spanish Blind. *Journal of European Public Policy.* June, 2: 2.

Garvia, R. 1996. The Professional Blind in Spain. *Work, Employment and Society*, Vol. 10, 3. September.

Gerra, L. L., Dorfman, S., Plaue, E., Schlackman, S. & Workman, D. 1995. Functional Communication as a Means of Decreasing Self-Injurious Behavior: A Case Study. *Journal of Visual Impairment and Blindness.* 89(4), pp. 343-348.

Gooch, A. 1991. Troubles Hit Spain's Empire of the Blind. *The Independent Newspaper*, June 8. London, England.

Goffman, E. 1963. *Stigma; Notes on the Management of Spoiled Identity.* Englewood Cliffs, NJ: Prentice-Hall.

Guide to ONCE with an introduction by José MaArroyo-Zarzosa. 1992. Published by the Social Service Department of ONCE, Madrid, Spain

Gwaltney, J. L. 1970. *The Thrice Shy.* Columbia University Press, NY.

Hill, M. M., Dodson-Burk, B., Fox, J. & Hill, E. W. 1995. An Infant Sonicguide Intervention Program for a Child with a Visual Disability. *Journal of Visual Impairment and Blindness.* 89(4), pp. 329-336.

Hull, J. M. 1990. *Touching the Rock: An Experience of Blindness.* New York: Pantheon Books.

ILO Regional Office for Asia and the Pacific Bangkok, 1994. *Towards Equalizing Opportunities for Disabled People in Asia: A Guide.*

Institutional Investor. 1993. International Edition. February, p. 16.

International Labor Standards on Vocational Rehabilitation: Guidelines for Implementation. 1984. ILO, Geneva, Switzerland.

Irwin, R. 1943. Why Rehabilitation of the Blind is a Function of a Special Agency for the Blind. *Outlook for the Blind,* p. 37 (10).

Isiko, N. 1993. Uganda and the Institutional Development Project. *The World Blind,* July - December. Madrid, Spain.

Jernigan, K. 1970. *Blindness - The Myth and the Image.* Reprinted in *Walking Alone and Marching Together,* pp. 289-299. Baltimore, MD: National Federation of the Blind.

Jernigan, K. 1996. Blindness: Handicap or Characteristic? *The World Blind,* Number 13, July.

Johnson, T. J. 1967. *Professions and Power.* London: MacMillan.

Kaufman, James M. and Hallahan, Daniel. 1995. *The Illusion of Full Inclusion.* Pro-Ed Inc., Austin, Texas.

Kazdin, Alan E. 1982. *Single-Case Research Designs.* New York, Oxford University Press.

Klee, K. (Ed.) 1993. *Institutional Investor,* February.

Koestler, F. A. 1976. *The Unseen Minority: A Social History of Blindness in America.* New York: David McKay.

Larson, M. S. 1977. *The Rise of Professionalism: A Sociological Analysis.* Berkely, CA: University of California Press.

Laws for the Protection of Citizens with Disabilities. 1990. Beijing: Government document.

Lazaro, R. 1993. ONCE's Social Services. Paper presented at the *International Expert Meeting on Library Services for the Visually Handicapped* in Barcelona, Spain. Paper available at ONCE.

Lowenfield, B. 1975. *The Changing Status of the Blind: From Separation to Integration.* Springfield, IL: Charles C. Thomas - Publisher, Bannerstone House.

MacKenzie, C. & Flowers, W. 1947. *Blindness in China.* Rochester, Kent, England: Stanhope Press Limited.

Mallory, Bruce L. Changing Beliefs About Disability in Developing Countries: Historical Factors and Sociocultural Variables. *Traditional and Changing Views of Disability in Developing Societies: Causes, Consequences, Cautions* (pp. 1-24). Ed. by Woods, D. Published by International Exchange of Experts and Information in Rehabilitation.

Martinéz, H. 1989. Trends in Rehabilitation Services for the Blind and Visually Impaired Within the Spanish National Organization of the Blind. Paper presented at *International Mobility Conference*, Netherlands. Paper available at ONCE.

Matras, J. 1990. *Dependency, Obligations and Entitlements.* Englewood Cliffs, NJ: Prentice-Hall.

Matson, F. 1990. *Walking Alone Marching Together: A History of the Organized Blind Movement in the United States, 1940-1990.* Baltimore, Maryland: The National Federation of the Blind.

Mettler, R. 1987. Blindness and Managing the Environment. *Journal of Visual Impairment and Blindness, 81*(10), pp. 476-481.

Mindes, J. 1991. A Study of Bilateral, Multicultural and International Voluntary Efforts to Help China Rehabilitate People with Disabilities. Unpublished paper, the International Exchange of Expertise and Information Rehabilitation Institute, Institute for Disabilities, University of New Hampshire, Durham.

Mpiriwe, D. & Diri-Baba, M. 1997. Issues Affecting Blind Women in the Rehabilitation Process. Published by the *World Blind Union*, Institutional Development Project (IDP). Watertown, Massachusetts.

Nagi, S. Z. Disability Concepts and Implications for Programs. Ed.by Gary Albrecht. *Cross-National Rehabilitation Policies.* Beverly Hills, CA: Sage.

Nicholls, R. An Examination of Some Traditional African Attitudes Toward Disability. *Traditional and Changing Views of Disability in Developing Societies: Causes, Consequences, Cautions.* Ed. by Woods, D. Published by International Exchange of Experts and Information in Rehabilitation.

Parish, W. & White, M. 1978. *Village and Family in Contemporary China.* Chicago: University of Chicago Press.

Patton, M. 1980. *Qualitative Evaluations Methods.* Beverly Hills, CA: Sage.

Pava, W. S. 1994. Visually Impaired Persons Vulnerability to Sexual and Physical Assault. *Journal of Visual Impairment and Blindness, 88*(2), pp. 103-112.

Pierce, B. 1994. Are Specialized Educational Settings for Children with Disabilities Immoral? *Braille Monitor*, February, pp. 71-79.

Reuters Limited, Reuters Financial Service. 1996. Venezuela Sells 15 Percent of Isla Bonita to Spain's ONCE, December 17.

Rosenfield, I. 1993. *The Strange, Familiar and Forgotten: An Anatomy of Consciousness.* New York: Vintage Books.

Rousseau, J. 1979/1762. *Emile on Education.* A. Bloom (Trans.) New York: Basic Books.

Rowland, W. P. 1985. *Being Blind in the World.* Pretoria, South Africa: Canterbury Book Printers.

Rowland, W. P. 1993. Making Life in a Rural Community a Quality Experience. *The World Blind,* July - December. Madrid, Spain.

Safford, P. & Safford, E. 1996. *A History of Childhood and Disability.* New York: Teachers College Press.

Salisbury, H. 1992. *The New Emperors: China in the Era of Mao and Deng.* Boston: Little, Brown.

Sangyeon, K. 1994. Fortune Tellers in Korea. *The World Blind,* No. 11: January - June.

Schama, S. 1989. *Citizens.* New York: Vintage Press.

Scharpf, Cordelia. 1996. Education of the Blind in the Peoples Republic of China: Attending Classes in Seven Schools for the Blind and Meeting Blind Chinese Women. The *ICEVH Educator,* July 4:2.

Schroeder, F. K. 1994. Expectations: The Critical Factor in the Education of Blind Children. *Braille Monitor,* February, pp.101-107.

Scott, R. A. 1967. The Factory as a Social Service Organization: Goal Displacement in Workshops for the Blind. *Social Problems, 15* (2), pp. 160-175.

Scott, R. A. 1969. *The Making of Blind Men.* Hartford, Ct: Connecticut Printers, Inc.

Sentumbwe, N. 1993. Understanding Blind/Sighted Relationships in Uganda. *The World Blind.* Madrid, Spain.

Siane, Lamin. 1997. Personal correspondence. October.

Sokolonska, M. et al. Creation and Removal of Disability as a Social Category: The Case of Poland. Ed. by Gary Albrect. Cross-National Rehabilitation Policies. Beverly Hills, CA: Sage.

Strauss, R. 1966. Social Change and the Rehabilitation Concept. *Sociology and Rehabilitation.* Ed. by M. B. Sussman. Chicago: American Sociological Association.

Stuckey, Kenneth A. 1996. Nearly Two Hundred Years of the European Influence o the Education of the Blind in America: How Were These Connections Made? First International Conference on *The Blind in History - The History of the Blind,* Copenhagen, October 6.

Sunquist, M. E., Montgomery, G. G. & Storm, G. L. 1969. Movements of a Blind Raccoon. *Journal of Mammology,* 50 (1), pp. 145-147.

Tawney, J. W. & Gast, D. L. 1984. *Single Subject Research in Special Education.* Columbus, OH: Charles E. Merrill Publishing Co.

tenBroek, J. 1956. Within the Grace of God, in *New Outlooks for the Blind,* 50, pp. 328-335.

tenBroek, J. 1962. The Character and Function of Sheltered Workshops. *The Blind American.* May, Volume II.

The Financial Times Limited. 1992. UAP Signs Agreement with ONCE to Sell a Range of Insurance Policies. World Corporate Insurance Report, February 14.

Thylefors, B. 1997. The Challenge of Combating Blindness in Africa. IAPB. Number 21, January.

Tovar, J. 1997. Personal interview at the ONCE headquarters in Madrid. At age 86 Tovar is still an active member of ONCE.

Tuttle, D. 1984. *Self-Esteem and Adjusting to Blindness: The Process of Responding to Life's Demands.* Springfield, IL: Charles C. Thomas.

Vaughan, C. E. & Vaughan, J. 1987. Sex Education of Blind Children Re-Examined. *Journal of Visual Impairment and Blindness.* March, pp. 95-98.

Vaughan, C. E. 1988. Self-Determination of Blind Workers in Chinese Guilds. *Braille Monitor.*

Vaughan, C. E. 1993. People-First Language: An Unholy Crusade. *Braille Monitor,* August, pp. 868-870.

Vaughan, C. E. 1993. *The Struggle of Blind People for Self Determination: The Dependency Rehabilitation Conflict: Empowerment in the Blindness Community.* Springfield, IL: Charles C. Thomas.

Vaughan, C. E. & Vaughan, J. 1994. "The Decline in Autonomy for Blind Workers in China." *RE:View.* Spring, XXVI, N. 1: 41-46.

Vaughan, C. E. and Zhang, C. 1996. The Impact of Modernization on Higher Education in China. *International Sociology.* Beverly Hills, CA: Sage.

Vaughan, C. E. 1997. Why Accreditation Failed Agencies Serving the Blind and Visually Impaired. *Journal of Rehabilitation,* January, February, March, pp. 7 - 14.

Vaughan, T., Reynolds, L. and Sjoberg, G. 1993. *A Critique of Contemporary American Sociology.* New York: General Hall, Inc.

Weber, M. 1951. *Religion of China: Confucianism and Taoism.* Glencoe, IL: Free Press.

Weber, M. 1978/1920. *Economy and Society.* G. Roth, Trans. New York: Bedminster.

Webson, A. 1997. *Empowerment of the Blind: A Handbook for Organizations of and for the Blind and Visually Impaired.* Hilton/Perkins Program, Watertown, Massachusetts.

Webson, A. 1997. Telephone conversation on May 27.

World Health Organization Onchocerciasis Expert Committee. 1995. "Onchocerciasis (or River Blindness) Control."

Wright, Beatrice A. 1988.

Zhang, N. 1990. Blind Physiotherapists in China. *The ICEVH Educator.* July, 3: 2.

Zurita, P. 1994. The Originality of the Spanish Model. *The World Blind, 11:* 15.

Zurita, P. 1997. Personal correspondence.

INDEX

A

AAWP (*see American Association of workers for the Blind*)

Adventitiously blind, 17

AER (*see Association for Education and Rehabilitation of the Blind and Visually Impaired*)

AFB (*see American Foundation for the Blind*)

Africa

blindness, 119-144

economic development, 119

First African Forum on Rehabilitation, 36

Gambia, 132, 133

Ghana, 137, 138

human rights of blind and visually impaired, 140, 141, 142, 143

visually impaired, 142, 143, 144

international cooperation, 129

Uganda, 135, 136, 137

African Forum on Rehabilitation, 128

African Union of the Blind (AFUB), 131

AFUB (*see African Union of the Blind*)

Agencies, 31, 33, 34, 35, 99, 100, 101, 102, 103, 104, 105, 106, 107, 108

harmful behavior, 33, 34, 35

social context of development, 101, 102, 103, 104, 105, 106, 107, 108

Albrecht, G., 33, 97

Almshouse, 96

American Association of Workers for the Blind (AAWP) Proceedings, 97

American Foundation for the Blind, 35, 101, 102, 105

Talking Books Program, 102, 105

American Council of the Blind, 64

Americans With Disabilities Act, 109

Ancient Greece, 89, 90

Anido, Martiez, 170

Apartheid (South Africa), 139

Association for the Education and Rehabilitation of the Blind and Visually Impaired (AER), 107

The Association of Persons with Severe Handicaps (TASH), 110

Asylums, 37, 93, 94

B

Barlow, J.M., 62

Being Blind in the World, 24

Best practice, 61, 62

Bentzen, B.L., 62

Biography of Tso, 145

BLIND Inc. (*see Blind Learning in New Dimensions, Inc.*)

Blind Learning in New Dimensions, Inc. (BLIND, Inc.), 107

"Blind massage", 145, 148, 149, 161, 162

Blind People: The Private and Public Life of Sightless Israelis, 53, 54

Blindness,

and consciousness, 55, 56, 57, 58, 59, 60

and culture, 8

and dependence, 23

and managing the environment, 75-87

and the New World Order, 36-39

as a characteristic of individuals, 40-50

as a learned social role, 29

consequences in relationships, 19, 21, 22

cross-cultural perspectives on, 3-8

cultural origins of, 89, 90, 91, 92, 93

false stereotypes of, 9

folk opinions of, 28, 29

historical and cultural influences, 54

in Africa, 119-144

Gambia, 132, 133

Ghana, 137, 138

South Africa, 139, 140

Sub-Saharan, 10

Uganda, 135, 136, 137
Zambia, 138, 139
in ancient China, 145, 146, 147
in antiquity, 89, 90
in China, 11, 145-166
in Costa Rica, 192
in less economically developed countries,
    10
in Mexico
    Mexican Village, 25-27
    in the Middle Kingdom (China), 144-146
    in The People's Republic of China, 147-
    166
in Spain, 11, 12, 24, 167-194
in the United States, 24, 31, 89-118
manufacturing ideas about, 51-87
organized responses to, 8, 9
phenomenology of, 8, 17-20
political context, 39, 40
prevention, 162, 188
producing images of, 51
psychological opinions of, 28, 29
social and cultural arrangements
    China, 155, 156, 157
    United States, 155, 156, 157
social and cultural perspectives, 17-50
social context, 27, 28
social interaction, 28-32
Braille, 95, 108, 131, 160, 162, 171, 188,
    189
    literacy, 111-118, 163
    shortage of in Africa, 130
Braille, Louis, 93
The Braille Monitor, 108
Buckley, S., 136
Bullington, J., 22
Bureaucratic structure, 6, 33
Burges, John, 146, 147
Burns, T., 176
Bush, George, 36
Busk, P.L., 73

C
Canadian National Institute for the Blind
    (CNIB), 126
Carter, President Jimmy, 151
Case Study, 70, 42, 73, 74
Cataract, 119, 159
Centro Bibliográfico y Cultural (Madrid,
    Spain), 177

Centro de Produccion Bibliográfico
    (Barcelona, Spain), 177
Centro Protectivo e Instructor de Ciegos
    (Spain), 169
Chan, G., 162
The Changing Status of the Blind, 89
Charities, 91
Children
    parental involvement in education, 118
    trends in education, 108-113
China (The Middle Kingdom and The
    People's Republic of China), 145-166
    blind population, 150
    disabilities, 158
    education of blind women and girls, 163-
    166
    First Five Year Plan for Disabled
    People, 11, 149
    guilds of blind workers, 11, 145
    modern era, 147-166
    new laws to protect people with disabilities,
    160-163
    social and cultural arrangements for blind
    people, 155-157
    social humanism, 161
China Disabled Persons' Association, 151
China Disabled Persons Federation (CDPF),
    162
China Welfare Fund for the Handicapped,
    151
China Communist Party, 39, 147, 148
Christoffel Blindenmission (Germany), 35,
    129, 162
Civil Rights Movement (U.S.), 109
Clemens, Samual, 100
Clinical evidence, 55
    "fundamental negative bias" in, 56
(CNIB) (*see Canadian National Institute for the
    Blind*)
Coleman, D.M., 98
Colorado Center for the Blind (U.S.), 107
Colors
    experience of, 21
    perception of, 19
"Common sense", 62
Comparative research, 73
Confucius, 145
Congenitally blind, 17
Cooperation
    international, 129

Pan-Africa, 130-132

Coordinadora Estatel de Minusvalidos Fisicos (CEMFE), 179, 180

Costa Rica, 192
blind workforce, 192

Cultural Revolution (1966-1976) (People's Republic of China), 148, 161

Culture
definition of, 8, 23, 24

D

Danish Association of the Blind, 138

Deng Pu Fang, 11, 150, 151, 157, 162

Deng Xiao Ping, 11, 39, 149, 150, 157

Dependency, 30

Deshen, S., 53, 54

Deuteronomy, 27:18, 90

Diderot, 92

Diri-Baba, M., 127, 128

Disabled People's Federation (People's Republic of China), 160

Disabilities,
in the People's Republic of China, 151, 158, 159, 160, 161, 162, 163
Organization Nacional de Ciegos Espanoles (ONCE) programs for people with physical disabilities, 177-181

Disibilities Education Act (IDEA) (U.S.), 109

Disability
benefits, 39
categories, 39
rates, 40

Domination and Subordination
patterns of, 7

Duff-Brown, B., 121

Duran, Miguel, 181, 182

E

Economic development, 119, 120, 121

Education, 108, 109, 110, 111, 112, 113, 117, 118, 159, 163, 183, 184, 185, 186, 187

Education for All Handicapped Children Act of 1975 (U.S.), 109, 117

The Educator, 163

Elizabethan Poor Laws of 1601, 91

Employment, 9, 54, 99, 100, 160, 161, 162, 163, 176, 177, 192, 193

Employment rate for blind people in Spain, 176, 177

Empowerment and Human Rights of Blind and Visually Impaired Persons in Africa, 140-144

The Empowerment of the Blind, 136

Enlightenment, 92, 168

Equal opportunity, 54

Equerra, Mr., 173

Experimental design, 62, 72

Expert knowledge, 62

F

Farrell, G., 94, 95

Fairbank, J., 146

Feagin, R., 72

Federation Hispanica de Ciegos (Spanish Federation of the Blind), 170

Federal Board of Vocational Education, 101

Fefoame, Gertrude, 131

Ferrell, K.A., 65, 66, 67, 72

Financial Times, 181

First African Forum on Rehabilitation, 36

First Five Year Plan (People's Republic of China), 149, 157-161

Fisher, John Dix, 93

Flowers, W., 146

Folk opinions, 19, 28

Foucault, Michel, 14

Franco, General, 11, 171

French, R.S., 54, 146

Fryer, G., 147

Full inclusion, 37

"Fundamental negative bias", 56

Future Reflections, 108

G

Gambia (Africa), 132, 133

Gambia Organization for the Visually Impaired (GOVI0, 132, 133

Garmezy, N., 70

Garvia, Roberto, 35, 168, 169, 170, 172, 173, 174, 175, 178, 179, 180

Gast, D.L., 73

Gender, 126, 127, 128, 163, 164, 165, 166

Gerra, L., 62

Ghana (Africa), 137, 138

Ghana Association of the Blind, 138

Ghana Society for the Blind (GSB), 137

Goffman, E., 13

GOVI (*see Gambia Organization for the Visually Impaired*)

Greece (*see Ancient Greece*)

GSB (*see Ghana Society for the Blind*)

Guilds, 11, 91, 145, 167

Gwaltney, J.L., 25, 27

H

Hallahan, Daniel, 110
Han Dynasty, 145
Hauy, Valentin, 92, 93
Hellen Keller International, 35
Hill, M.M., 64, 65, 66, 72, 73
Hilton-Perkins International Program (U.S.),
    36, 129
Holt, Edith, 100
Holt, Winifred, 100
Hong Kong Society for the Blind, 162
Hope Deferred, 98
Hospitals, 90, 91
Howe, Samual Gridley, 10, 93, 94, 95, 109
Hull, John, 55, 56, 57, 58
Human rights, 140-144
Human subjects, 74
Humanistic concerns, 151
Hypothetico-deductive methodology, 62

I

IDP (*see International Development Project*)
IEP (*see Individual Education Plan*)
Illiteracy, 38
    (*see also Literacy and Braille literacy*)
ILO (*see International Labor Organization*)
IMF (*see International Monetary Fund*)
The Independent of London, 182
Individual Education Plan (IEP), 117
Infama, 140
INGO (*see International Non-Government
    Organization*)
L' Institute National Pour les Sueugles
    (*see The National Institute for Blind Youth*)
Institutional Investor, 181
Interdisciplinary research, 71, 73
Internal validity, 73
International cooperation, 187-189
International Development Project (IDP),
    129
International Labor Organization (ILO), 36,
    38, 129
International Monetary Fund (IMF), 36, 129
International Non-Government Organi-
    zation (INGO), 120
Internet, 70
Irwin, Robert B., 101, 102, 105
Isiko, Nelson, 135

J

Jernigan, Kenneth, 12, 40
    condensed version of his article "Blindness:
    Handicap or Characteristic?", 41-50
Johnson, T.J., 35
Journal of Mammology, 60
Journal of Rehabilitation, 107
Journal of Visual Impairment and Blindness
    (JVIB, 62, 63, 64, 72, 73, 75
JVIB (*see Journal of Visual Impairment and
    Blindness*)

K

Karlsson, 22
Kauffman, James M., 110
Kazdin, A., 71
Keller, Helen, 28, 105
Klein, Johann Wilhelm, 93
Knowledge
    argumentation, 72
    "common sense", 62
    empirical scientific, 60
    epistemological questions, 72
    expert, 62
    historical perspective, 72
    human reason, 72
    scientific, 51, 52, 62
    theoretical assumptions, 72
Koestler, F.A., 105

L

Labor unions, 99
La Forge, Jan, 12
Language
    politically correct, 12-15
    preferred, 12-15
Larson, M.S., 34
Latin America
    Organization National de Ciegos,
    Espanoles economic support, 187, 188,
    189
Laws
    news laws to protect people with disabili-
    ties in the People's Republic of China,
    160-163
Leviticus 19:14, 90
Literacy
    Braille literacy, 111-118, 163
    (*see also Illiteracy*)

Literature reviews
  in scientific research, 65-69
Lottery
  in Spain, 170-184;, 190, 191, 192, 193, 194
Louisiana Center for the Blind, 107
Lowenfeld, Berthold, 30, 89, 90, 91, 92, 93, 94, 95, 102, 109
Luck, Lawrence, 112
Lu T'a I, 145

M

Madrid School for the Blind (Spain), 169
Mainstream programs, 139
Mainstreaming, 37, 108, 109, 110, 116, 159, 186
Makenzie, C., 146
The Making of Blind Men, 28, 29, 30, 31, 32
Mallory, Bruce L., 150
Mao Tse Tung, 30
Mark Twain (*see Samuel Clemens*)
Masquete, Antonio Vicente, 176
Matras, J., 39
Matson, Floyd, 98
Maurer, Marc, 113
Merck Pharmaceutical Company, 122
Mettler, Richard, 72, 75
Mexico
  blindness in a Mexican village, 25-27
  San Pedro Yolox, 25-27
Middle Ages, 146
Mindes, J., 162
Mondaca, Rafael, 188
Mpirirwe, D., 127, 128
Multivariate parametic analysis, 62

N

NAC (*see National Accreditation Council for Agencies Serving the Blind and Visually Handicapped*)
Nagi, S.Z., 40
National Accreditation Council for Agencies Serving the Blind and Visually Handicapped (NAC), 107
National Federation of the Blind (NFB), 7, 10, 12, 33, 54, 99, 103, 107, 113, 117
  The Braille Monitor, 108
  Future Reflections, 108
  The Voice of the Diabetic, 108
National Federation of the Blind (Spain), 169

National Industries for the Blind (NIB), 99, 101, 102
National Institute of General Medical Science, 60
National Institute for Blind Youth, 93
Natural science model, 52
Natural science paradigm, 62
Nebraska Services for the Blind, 75
Neurology, 55
New England Asylum for the Blind, 99, 100
New World Order, 36-39
New York Association for the Blind, 99, 100
New York Institute for the Education of the Blind, 93
NGO (*see Non-governmental organizations*)
Nicholls, R., 123, 124
NIB (*see National Industries for the Blind*)
Nkrumah, Kwame, 137
Non-governmental organizations, 6, 36, 38, 51, 128, 129, 188
Norwegian Association of the Blind and Partially Sighted, 131

O

Occupations, 145, 146, 147, 148, 149, 150, 172, 173, 174
ONCE (*see Organización Nacional de Ciegos Españoles*)
Onchocerciasis, 119, 121
Opthalmologists, 122
Opium War, 32
Organized Blind Movement (U.S.), 37, 38
Organizacíon Nacional de Ciegos Españoles (ONCE), 11, 12, 24, 35
  educational services, 183-187
  international cooperation, 187
  physical disabilities programs, 177-181
  rehabilitation services, 183-197
Orum, H.M., 72

P

Parish, W., 148
Patriarchism, 128
Patton, M., 62, 71, 74
Pava, W.S., 64
Parkins School for the Blind, 10, 28, 93, 94, 129
Phenomenology
  of blindness, 17-20

Philanthropists, 100
Pierce, B., 37
Plato, 90
Politically correct language, 12-15
Poor relief tax of 1554, 91
Poorhouses, 168
Positivism, 71, 72, 74
PRODIECU, 178, 179, 180
Professional development, 188
Professions, 99-108
Professions and Power, 35
Psychological opinions
  about blindness, 28, 29
Public Health education, 122

Q
Qualitative research, 71, 72, 73
Quantitative research, 62

R
Racoons
  critique of research on blind racoons, 60,
  61
Randolph-Shepard Act of 1936, 101
Recorded books, 130
Regular Education Initiative (REI), 110
Rehabilitation, 5, 6, 7, 9, 33, 38, 39, 40, 71,
  98, 99, 100, 137, 138, 140, 149, 151, 152,
  183, 184, 185, 186, 187
REI (*see Regular Education Initiative*)
Reischaver, E., 146
Religion
  Judaism, 90
  Christianity, 90
  Islam, 90
Religious organizations, 95, 96
Representativeness, 62, 63, 64
Research design, 64, 65
Reuters, 181
Rivera, Primo de, 170
Roman Empire, 90
Rosenfield, Israel, 55, 56, 57, 58, 60
Rousseux, Emile, 92
Rowland, William, 17, 18, 19, 20, 21, 23, 24,
  25, 27, 126, 139, 140
Royal Commonwealth Society for the Blind
  (Now Sight Savers), 137
Royal Institute for the Blind, 162

S
Safford, E., 108
Safford, P., 108
Salisbury, H., 148, 151
Salvation Army, 96
Sample size, 62, 63, 64, 74
Sampling technique, 74
San Pedro Yolox, 25-27
Sangyeon, 145
Satrustegui, Ignacio, 176
Scharpf, Cordelia, 163
School for Deaf and Blind Children in Xi'an,
  152
Schools for the Blind, 92, 93, 94, 95, 96, 97,
  98, 99, 130, 138
Schroeder, Fred, 37
Schuster, Clara Shaw, 67
Science
  as the highest form of knowledge, 52
  assumptions of, 52
  natural science model, 52
  "objectivity", 52
  scientific method, 52
Scientific investigation
  unit of analysis, 69
Scientific knowledge, 52, 62
Scientific methodology, 9
Scientific methods, 51, 52, 60
Scientific research
  internal validity, 73
  methods, 73
  qualitative, 71
  "narrow focus", 71
Scott, Robert, 28, 29, 30, 31, 32, 33, 34, 97,
  103, 154
Self-determination, 8
*Self-esteem and Adjusting to Blindness: The
  Process of Responding to Life's Demands*, 31-32,
  56
Sentumbwe, Nayinda, 126
Sex education, 67, 68, 69
Sexual relationships, 126, 127, 128
Sheltered workshops, 95-99, 102, 149
Shih K'uang, 145, 146
Siane, Lamin, 133
Sight Savers International (U.K.), 35, 129,
  130, 137
Single subject designs, 70

Smith-Fess Act, 100
Social context, 27-28
Social control, 6, 35
Social and cultural arrangements for blind
  people, 155-157
Social inequality, 126
Social interaction, 28-32
Social learning, 29
Social role, 29
Social Security Administration (U.S.), 103
Social Security (U.S.), 10, 102
Socialist humanism
  in the People's Republic of China, 161
Socialization, 28, 29, 30
Sokolonska, M., 40
Solon of Athens, 90
South Africa, 139-140
South Africa National Council for the Blind
  (SANCB), 139, 140
  Infama, 140
South African Society for the Blind, 20
Spain
  blindness in, 167-194
  employment rate of blind, 176, 177
  job training programs, 173
  occupations of the blind, 172, 173, 174
  lottery, 170-194
  lottery ticket sellers, 172, 173, 174
  Organization Nacional de Ciegos
    Espanoles (ONCE), 11, 12, 24, 35, 177,
    178, 179, 180, 181, 183, 184, 185, 186, 187
  PORDIECU, 178, 179, 180
Spanish Civil War, 171
Spanish Federation of the Blind, 170, 171
Spanish National Organization of the Blind,
  167
Special education, 9, 108
Ssu Song Ming, 145
The Strange, Familiar and Forgotten, 55
Sullivan, 28
Sunquist, M.E., 60
Supplemental Security Income of 1974
  (U.S.), 103
Stuckey, Kenneth A., 93
Symbolic language, 21

T
Talking books, 188, 189
Talking Books Program, 102, 105
Tape Aids for the Blind of South Africa, 130

TASH (*see The Association of Persons with Severe
  Handicaps*)
Tawney, J.W., 73
Tembo, B.K., 139
tenBroek, Jacobus, 33, 95, 98, 103
Tennessee Commission for the Blind, 98
Tennessee School for the Blind, 98
Thylefors, B., 122, 125
Touching the Rock, 55, 56, 57, 58
Tovar, Javier Gutierrez de, 171, 174
Toward Equalizing Opportunities, 38
"Trauma of blindness", 31, 32
Trachoma, 119, 122
Tso Chiu, 145
Tuttle, Dean, 31, 32, 55
Twain, Mark (*see Clemens, Samuel*)
Tzu, Hsia, 145

U
Uganda Organization of the Blind, 11
Uganda National Association of the Blind,
  128, 135, 136
Unit of analysis, 69
United Nations, 36, 129, 152
University of Minnesota, 60
United States Atomic Energy Commission,
  60
United States
  American Foundation for the Blind (AFB),
    35
  blindness in, 89-118
  collective interests, 31
  federal government services to the blind,
    100, 101
  Federal Vocational Education Board, 101
  Great Depression, 102
  organized blind movement, 37-38
  social and cultural arrangements for blind
    people, 155, 156, 157
  Smith-Fess Act, 100
  state government services to the blind,
    100, 101
  veterns, 100, 101
  Veterns Administration, 101
  Works Project Administration, 102

V
Vaughan, C. Edwin, 14, 33, 34, 35, 67,
  91, 95, 105, 107, 108, 145, 158
Vaughan, JoAn, 67, 89, 91, 145

Vaughan, T., 52
Veterans, 100, 101
Veterans Administration (U.S.), 101
Voltaire, 92

W
WBU (*see World Blind Union*)
Weber, Max, 6, 33, 146
Webson, Aubrey, 36, 128, 136
WHO (*see World Health Organization*)
Whyte, M., 148
Wilson, President, 100
Women
  blind in People's Republic of China, 163,
    164, 165, 166
Workhorse, 96
World Bank, 151
The World Blind, 40, 188
World Blind Union (WBU), 129, 187, 188
World Health Organization (WHO), 36, 39,
  120, 123, 129

World War I, 100, 101
World War II, 36, 73, 102
Wright Beatrice, A., 56
Wunder, Gary, 58
  response to John Hull's *Touching the Rock,*
    58-60

X
Xerophalmia, 119, 122
Xeuodochium, 90
Xi'an Foreign Language University, 152
Xu Bailum, 63

Z
Zabala, Kepa Conde, 188
Zambia (Africa), 138-139
Zhang, N., 149
Zurita, P., 171, 172, 176, 177, 181, 183, 187